Monica :
enjoy !
Jo Ann

Help! My Underwear is Shrinking!

Jo Ann Hattner, MPH, RD • Ann Coulston, MS, RD
E. Michael Goodkind, BA

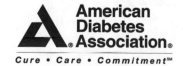
American
Diabetes
Association®
Cure • Care • Commitment℠

Director, Book Publishing, John Fedor; *Associate Director, Consumer Books,* Sherrye Landrum, *Editor,* Abe Ogden; *Associate Director, Book Production,* Peggy M. Rote; *Composition,* Circle Graphics, Inc.; *Cover Design,* Koncept Inc.; *Printer,* Port City Press.

Printed in the United States of America
1 3 5 7 9 10 8 6 4 2

∞ The paper in this publication meets the requirements of the ANSI Standard Z39.48-1992 (permanence of paper).

ADA titles may be purchased for business or promotional use or for special sales. To purchase this book in large quantities, or for custom editions of this book with your logo, contact Lee Romano Sequeira, Special Sales & Promotions, at the address below, or at LRomano@diabetes.org or 703-299-2046.

American Diabetes Association
1701 North Beauregard Street
Alexandria, Virginia 22311

Library of Congress Cataloging-in-Publication Data

Hattner, Jo Ann, 1941–
    Help! : my underwear is shrinking / Jo Ann Hattner, Ann Coulston, Mike Goodkind.
        p. cm.
    Includes index.
    ISBN 1-58040-179-1 (pbk. : alk. paper)
        1. Non-insulin-dependent diabetes—Diet therapy. I. Coulston, Ann M. II. Goodkind, Mike, 1943– III. Title.

RC662.18.H38 2003
616.4'620654—dc21

                                                                    2003048071

Contents

CHAPTER ONE

My Underwear
Is Shrinking!

L ike some 5 million of the 16 million Americans who
unknowingly suffer from type 2 (adult-onset) diabetes,
Tiffany felt no symptoms. She felt no pain, no ill effects,
no indication that something was wrong. She did, however,
feel that she had developed a few, well . . . clumps.

"My underwear is shrinking!" she screamed one evening
as she looked in the mirror. The sight of her disappearing
underpants sent a jolt through her ample body. Her husband's increasing indifference as she slid under the covers
wasn't helping much either. She realized she needed a change.

Tiffany had tried many diets in her 30-something years,
but despite what she thought were her best efforts, the love
handles continued to grow. Yet she was determined to make
another try, so she called her doctor.

When her doctor's receptionist asked what the problem
was, Tiffany replied, "I feel fine. I just need a diet."

Tiffany wasn't lying. She did feel fine. So when she came
for her appointment with Dr. Dillon, she was surprised at all
the health history questions his assistant, Carla, patiently
asked.

"What does my grandmother's health have to do with
anything?" Tiffany asked. "Grandma passed away years
ago." But Carla persevered, and Tiffany reluctantly went
along with what seemed a waste of time "just to get a diet."

When Dr. Dillon finally came into the room, he reminded Tiffany that her mother had been diagnosed with type 2
diabetes at age 52, and her maternal grandmother had died

1

of a stroke at age 72. He noted that diabetes typically runs in families, and that stroke is often a sign of diabetes.

"Tiffany, because of your family history, I think you should have a blood sugar test," the doctor said.

Tiffany still wanted her diet.

"But I'm only in my 30s, I don't have any symptoms, and all I want is to lose some weight," she protested.

But Dr. Dillon was firm. "First things first," he said.

At 8 A.M. the next morning, Tiffany drove to the lab for her fasting blood glucose test. She had done as she was told and hadn't eaten since the evening before at about 7:30, when she finished the last half of the donut her husband had left in the kitchen ("After all," she reasoned, "I won't be eating for quite awhile"). At the lab, the line was long and she had to wait an hour for her test. By the time she left, she was starving, so she stopped off and bought 2 bagels. She felt so healthy as she quickly scarfed them down—without any cream cheese or topping, just plain ole bagels. Well, there were some chocolate chips in one of them, but after all . . .

A few days later she got a call from Carla at the doctors office.

"Tiffany, we're going to need you to come back for some more tests."

"Did something go wrong?" Tiffany asked.

"Not exactly," replied Carla. "But we're going to need another fasting glucose test."

So, Tiffany went through the whole thing again. A week later Carla called again.

"Well, Tiff (Carla and Tiffany were friends from PTA), the lab results came back and I've got some good news and some bad news."

Tiffany wondered how there could be any good news if there was also bad news, so she just held her breath and waited for the worst.

But Carla was actually pretty cheery. "Well, your blood sugar is 130 milligrams per deciliter. Between 70 and 110 is considered normal. Also, just as you suspected, you could stand to lose a few pounds. To be specific your BMI—body mass index—is 28."

"What the heck are you talking about? Listen, Carla, I can handle it," Tiffany said impatiently. "So forget about this B-M-whatever stuff and tell me, how much do I weigh?"

"We use BMI," Carla patiently explained, "because it is a more helpful tool. If I knew your weight without knowing your height, I couldn't tell very much. For instance, 170 pounds would be a pretty lean weight for someone taller than 6 feet tall, but obese for someone only 5 feet tall. You're 5 foot 5, so your BMI of 28 is in the overweight range, and unfortunately, you are at a greater risk than normal for heart disease and diabetes. Besides your weight, Tiffany, we found that your blood pressure is running on the high side—130 over 80—and that's another health risk.

"At any rate, your blood glucose level means that you qualify for a diagnosis of type 2 diabetes. Some people call this adult-onset diabetes."

There was a pause on the phone before Carla continued.

"You see, Tiff, your body is making insulin, it just doesn't use it efficiently. Eating and weighing too much both make this condition worse. We call this insulin resistance. This is different than type 1 diabetes, which is much less common. Only about 10 percent of the people with diabetes, like Steve, Jackie's little boy, have that type. In type 1, the body doesn't make any insulin at all, so people who have that form of diabetes have to take insulin injections to stay alive."

Actually, Tiffany knew all this—except the part about young Steve having diabetes. She had gone through all of this when her mother was diagnosed with diabetes several years before, but she didn't have the heart to stop her friend from reminding her of the basic facts. What she really wanted to know was what could possibly be the good news Carla said was coming. And when the heck was she going to get her diet?

"In fact," Carla said downright happily, "the good news is you don't have to take insulin or any other medication, at

Body Mass Index Table

	Normal						Overweight					Obese					
BMI	19	20	21	22	23	24	25	26	27	28	29	30	31	32	33	34	35
Height (inches)							Body Weight (pounds)										
58	91	96	100	105	110	115	119	124	129	134	138	143	148	153	158	162	167
59	94	99	104	109	114	119	124	128	133	138	143	148	153	158	163	168	173
60	97	102	107	112	118	123	128	133	138	143	148	153	158	163	168	174	179
61	100	106	111	116	122	127	132	137	143	148	153	158	164	169	174	180	185
62	104	109	115	120	126	131	136	142	147	153	158	164	169	175	180	186	191
63	107	113	118	124	130	135	141	146	152	158	163	169	175	180	186	191	197
64	110	116	122	128	134	140	145	151	157	163	169	174	180	186	192	197	204
65	114	120	126	132	138	144	150	156	162	168	174	180	186	192	198	204	210
66	118	124	130	136	142	148	155	161	167	173	179	186	192	198	204	210	216
67	121	127	134	140	146	153	159	166	172	178	185	191	198	204	211	217	223
68	125	131	138	144	151	158	164	171	177	184	190	197	203	210	216	223	230
69	128	135	142	149	155	162	169	176	182	189	196	203	209	216	223	230	236
70	132	139	146	153	160	167	174	181	188	195	202	209	216	222	229	236	243
71	136	143	150	157	165	172	179	186	193	200	208	215	222	229	236	243	250
72	140	147	154	162	169	177	184	191	199	206	213	221	228	235	242	250	258
73	144	151	159	166	174	182	189	197	204	212	219	227	235	242	250	257	265
74	148	155	163	171	179	186	194	202	210	218	225	233	241	249	256	264	272
75	152	160	168	176	184	192	200	208	216	224	232	240	248	256	264	272	279
76	156	164	172	180	189	197	205	213	221	230	238	246	254	263	271	279	287

From the National Heart, Lung, and Blood Institute (NHLBI) of the National Institutes of Health's Obesity Education Initiative, launched Jan. 1991.

				Extreme Obesity														
36	37	38	39	40	41	42	43	44	45	46	47	48	49	50	51	52	53	54
								Body Weight (pounds)										
172	177	181	186	191	196	201	205	210	215	220	224	229	234	239	244	248	253	258
178	183	188	193	198	203	208	212	217	222	227	232	237	242	247	252	257	262	267
184	189	194	199	204	209	215	220	225	230	235	240	245	250	255	261	266	271	276
190	195	201	206	211	217	222	227	232	238	243	248	254	259	264	269	275	280	285
196	202	207	213	218	224	229	235	240	246	251	256	262	267	273	278	284	289	295
203	208	214	220	225	231	237	242	248	254	259	265	270	278	282	287	293	299	304
209	215	221	227	232	238	244	250	256	262	267	273	279	285	291	296	302	308	314
216	222	228	234	240	246	252	258	264	270	276	282	288	294	300	306	312	318	324
223	229	235	241	247	253	260	266	272	278	284	291	297	303	309	315	322	328	334
230	236	242	249	255	261	268	274	280	287	293	299	306	312	319	325	331	338	344
236	243	249	256	262	269	276	282	289	295	302	308	315	322	328	335	341	348	354
243	250	257	263	270	277	284	291	297	304	311	318	324	331	338	345	351	358	365
250	257	264	271	278	285	292	299	306	313	320	327	334	341	348	355	362	369	376
257	265	272	279	286	293	301	308	315	322	329	338	343	351	358	365	372	379	386
265	272	279	287	294	302	309	316	324	331	338	346	353	361	368	375	383	390	397
272	280	288	295	302	310	318	325	333	340	348	355	363	371	378	386	393	401	408
280	287	295	303	311	319	326	334	342	350	358	365	373	381	389	396	404	412	420
287	295	303	311	319	327	335	343	351	359	367	375	383	391	399	407	415	423	431
295	304	312	320	328	336	344	353	361	369	377	385	394	402	410	418	426	435	443

least not now. If you lose weight, you may never need to take meds. Dr. Dillon thinks you can be treated first with lifestyle modification. He wants you to try that for six months. After that, come on back, we'll run another blood test, and Dr. Dillon will evaluate your progress. Meanwhile, go see someone who can help you start making those lifestyle changes right away. Do you have any questions?"

Tiffany had about four hundred questions. She was overwhelmed and confused—this was a lot to take in for one phone call. She didn't know how she was supposed to feel. Where did she go from here? What did she need to do? Was this serious? Should she be worried about this? How could she fix this? Carla seemed so breezy and cheerful—maybe it was no big deal. Or maybe she was just softening the blow. Tiffany didn't know. In fact, Tiffany was starting to feel like there was *a lot* she didn't know. Where should see begin? What question should she ask first?

As it turns out, she wouldn't ask any questions at all. Just as she was about to start her barrage of queries, a loud crash shot through the house, followed shortly by whimpering and crying—her son had somehow just rammed his bike into the back door. Motherly instincts trumped self-preservation and Tiff abruptly ended her conversation with Carla. She hung up the phone and ran to the back door to make sure her kid was okay, BMIs and insulin resistance temporarily pushed to the back of her mind.

The First Move

The next day was Saturday. After eating the 3 individual-serving boxes of no-fat shredded wheat she'd picked up from the motel buffet on her last work trip, Tiffany pulled out her phone book and began looking in the yellow pages under "lifestyle" to find a consultant. Under lifestyle she found a few listings, including one with a small picture of a young lady who obviously had never needed a diet. This "consult-ant" was available 24 hours a day and would make something called outcalls for gentlemen. Tiffany suspected this probably wouldn't help either her diabetes or her diet.

A little discouraged, Tiffany started to look under the "consultants" listing. Unfortunately, before she could get too far her husband, Tom, told her they needed to get moving if they wanted to pick out that new dishwasher they'd been planning to buy.

So it was Monday morning before Tiffany got back to thinking about her diet, not to mention diabetes.

"My doctor says I should find a consultant to make lifestyle modifications," she told her fellow worker, Sue Ellen. "But I don't have a clue how to get started. And why can't Dr. Dillon just give me a diet?" It was then that Tiffany confided to Sue Ellen about her increasing weight—Sue Ellen tried to feign surprise—and about her diabetes.

Sue Ellen knew exactly what to say.

"Geez, honey, what you need is a nutritionist—a registered dietitian. They know all about lifestyle change and diabetes. They can help you focus and plan what you need to do for yourself. A good nutritionist can help flesh out what your doctor thinks you need to do." Sue Ellen noticed that Tiffany was giving her a how-do-you-know-all-this look. "My neighbor, Lorraine, also has diabetes. She went on a diet and lifestyle plan, and boy, does she look great. Let me find out the name of the person who helped her."

The next day at work, Sue Ellen handed Tiffany the phone number for a nutritionist named Joanne. She was a recognized professional, a registered dietitian, and member of the American Dietetic Association.

CHAPTER TWO

Getting Started

"I think I'm doing all the right things," Tiffany said, nearly in tears during her phone call to Joanne, the registered dietitian. "But I keep putting on pounds. They just creep up on me. I've been gaining weight now for about 5 years. And now my doctor says I have type 2 diabetes. He says my weight makes the diabetes worse. I know my health, my appearance, and somewhere down the line, maybe even my marriage all depend on what I can do to make, you know, lifestyle changes. Please. What can I do?"

"Don't worry, I understand," Joanne reassured her. "Come down and we'll talk. But before we can think about lifestyle modifications we have to find out what we're going to modify. When I understand a little bit more about you, I will help you develop a simple, positive healthy eating plan—customized just for you."

Tiffany felt a little more reassured as she walked into the office complex where Joanne worked. Since she was early enough for the appointment, she stopped at the Galaxy Dollar Coffee Store on the ground floor for one of her favorite specialty drinks, a white chocolate mocha with skim milk.

"Let's start with some questions about your habits," said Joanne.

Here we go with the questions, thought Tiffany. But it occurred to her that this may not be such a bad thing. Maybe, despite what thousands of magazine articles, books, and talk shows were spouting, a diet was a very personal

As you go through this book, you will be getting the step-by-step planning and assistance that the authors regularly provide to clients. This book is like having your own private lifestyle counselor by your side.

affair. If Dr. Dillon wouldn't just hand her a diet, how could she expect that a dietitian like Joanne would be any less thorough?

Joanne could almost feel Tiffany's frustration as her new client sat across the table and shared a few thoughts about her life.

"Joanne, is it diabetes that's making my weight so hard to control?"

"I don't think so," said Joanne. "So far I haven't gotten any indication that you are any different in your lifestyle or weight profile than my clients whose blood sugar is normal."

The two chatted more about Tiffany's habits. In addition to her family's history of diabetes, it turns out that Tiffany's father died of heart disease in his 60s, giving her one more risk factor—cardiac disease—and even more incentive to pursue a healthy diet.

Look at your own family history. Your medical team has probably talked to you about diabetes in your family, but remind yourself of other trends. If one or more close family members died relatively early of heart disease, it's a good idea to ask your doctor what you should do. Heart disease risk is increased in people with diabetes. Certainly a healthy diet will be a part of your overall prevention for this number-one killer of Americans—men and women.

Table 2-1. Family History

Complete the form by filling in names, medical conditions, and the approximate age the conditions occurred. For example: type 1 diabetes, type 2 diabetes, high blood pressure, heart disease (bypass or stroke), cancer (breast, colon, lung), and arthritis.

Paternal		Maternal	
Grandfather	Grandmother	Grandfather	Grandmother
_____	_____	_____	_____
_____	_____	_____	_____
_____	_____	_____	_____
_____	_____	_____	_____

Aunts	Father	Uncles	Aunts	Mother	Uncles
____	____	____	____	____	____
____	____	____	____	____	____
____	____	____	____	____	____
____	____	____	____	____	____

Siblings	Your name	Siblings
_____	_____	_____
_____	_____	_____
_____	_____	_____
_____	_____	_____

Joanne then asked a few questions about activity. Tiffany was certainly no athlete, but she did have a gym membership and lots of good intentions about exercising. This was a start. At least the intent was there. Joanne saw this as something they could address together a bit later.

A What? A Carbovore? Who, Me?

Tiffany was a responsible, conscientious person with a reasonable regard for her own health and diet. So what was going on? Joanne asked if any of the following statements applied to her.

While we wait for Tiffany's answers, ask yourself which of these statements applies to you.

- You eat lots of foods that you thought couldn't make you fat because they were nonfat or low fat and, therefore, healthy in your mind.
- Your most frequent food choices are foods with a high percentage of carbohydrates (carbs)—bread, potatoes, rice, grain, fruits (sorry about that), and of course, candy, chips, and sodas.
- In the morning you want only carbs—a muffin, cereal, toast, or pancakes. No bacon for you!
- You use carbs to pick you up in the midmorning (doughnuts or bagels) and in the afternoon (energy bars, candy bars, or sodas).
- You look for excuses to eat carbs. You wouldn't think of doing this alone, but at night you join your child in a bedtime snack of Frosty Frizzle Flake Cereal.
- You have convinced yourself that carbohydrates are healthy. For example, the frozen yogurt and chocolate sorbet are nonfat, so they aren't bad for you.

- You indulge in what you tell yourself are "healthy binges." You crave carbs and find yourself seeking out a bakery to buy a loaf of French bread, which you devour all by yourself.

This test is easy. How many apply to you?

After answering a resounding "yes" to every single situation, Tiffany seemed a little shocked. "I'm a carbovore!" she yelped.

"Well, Tiffany," said Joanne, "I think you are a good candidate for a diet plan we will customize for you. I call it Carbohydrate Countdown."

Tiffany was interested. This sounded different than the everyday low-fat plans she normally self-prescribed.

"Now, you called yourself a carbovore," continued Joanne. "Some people prefer carboholic. But whatever term you use, the reality is that carbs are the center of your food life. You, like millions of other people—mostly women, as it turns out—have been mentally programmed by simplified health messages, advertising, and even old Aunt Bea to think of fats as evil. It's not too much of a jump to think, that 'if fats are bad, then carbs are good.' And from there the logic follows that 'if carbs are good, I can eat as much as I want and stay healthy.' So when many people give up fats, they overcompensate by gobbling up carbs."

Tiffany was a little taken aback by how well Joanne had pegged her eating habits. She had always figured that if a food was fat-free, it was pretty much fair game. She'd never considered how carbs were figuring into her weight gain. But still, Joanne's plan sounded so different from what she'd been taught all of her life that she was a little skeptical. Plus, all of this talk about diabetes made her even more unsure.

"Joanne, I can relate to what you're saying about carbohydrates," Tiffany finally said. "But being diagnosed with diabetes has made me a little more conscious about my

health. I'm wondering how scientifically sound your diet
plan is."

"That's a valid concern," Joanne replied. "But not to
worry, there is indeed a scientific basis for Carbohydrate
Countdown. My recommendations are based on longstand-
ing agreements among health professionals. What I'll show
you is based on sound nutritional principles. For years, dietitians at Stanford University Medical Center have been using
and perfecting this diet for patients with diabetes. You've
probably heard this before, but it's worth repeating: There is
nothing different about nutrition for persons with type 2 diabetes who need to lose weight than for other people, except
that when your blood sugar is problematic, you need to follow those principles with extra care. And that's what we'll
be doing.

"This plan focuses on carbohydrates because we have
found that carbs are central to your cravings, and as I'm confident we'll see, your eating patterns as well. There are probably 2 underlying reasons for carb cravings; one scientific,
the other cultural.

"As for science, researchers are coming up with some
explanations about what is happening in your body. A craving for carbohydrates may occur because this food appears
to increase levels of a chemical that in turn increases levels of
serotonin, a natural brain chemical that has been found to
alter mood. Serotonin can produce a feeling of well-being if
it is present in the right quantity. It's an interesting theory,
and is certainly the basis for an interesting discussion. But
even if serotonin isn't responsible, I think it's safe to say that
at least some of our food cravings are responses to our bodies' fundamental chemical needs," Joanne said.

Tiffany's eyes were beginning to glaze over. Joanne
sensed she was starting to lose her. Time to shift gears.

"In any case—forget science for a moment—our society,
through advertising, popular culture, whatever, has programmed us to eat in ways that make it difficult to control
our weight."

Tiffany perked up. This programming stuff seemed to pique her interest.

"Tiffany, how often have you eaten a bit too much of a food item because it was advertised as 'fat-free?' I think deep in your heart you know that doesn't mean it will make YOU fat free . . ."

"But it sure makes me feel less guilty to eat it," Tiffany responded.

"Exactly," continued Joanne. "For many years we've been taught, 'Give up fat, and you'll do your heart a favor, avoid a number of killer cancers, and'—now here's the real myth—'you'll lose weight, too.'

"Certainly a low fat diet is important. *We are not advising you eat a high-fat diet.* But if you replace all of the fatty foods you give up with bagels, pasta, nonfat yogurt, fat-free ice cream, and other carbohydrate-packed foods, you won't win the weight-loss war. That's because you will have become a *carboholic*, or, as you liked to put it, a *carbovore*."

"I did try one of those high-protein, high-fat diets before, and I actually lost some weight," Tiffany recalled.

"But did you gain it back?" Joanne asked softly. "There is a built-in flaw in those diets, no matter how quickly they help you lose weight. When you restrict foods to lose weight, like you do on those specialty plans, you end up denying yourself essential foods and nutrients. Yes, you can regain some of these nutrients from supplements, but this is a tricky balance that is very hard to achieve. Most people simply don't have the time or skills to do this. Sooner or later, you are drawn back to carbs. Many of my clients are lapsed carboholics who have gained weight after completing a high-protein or similar specialty diet. To keep you from lapsing as well, my plan includes some new ingredients to help motivate you and help you stick to a diet and make . . .

". . . lifestyle modifications." Tiffany and Joanne said the last two words together.

"Tiffany, we have found that without lifestyle modifications, sticking with a diet is almost impossible. Diet and healthy eating have to be part of our lives—not extra baggage to carry around. We've learned that from years of experience."

"You keep saying 'we.' Who else are you talking about?" Tiffany asked.

"Well, I didn't come up with the Carbohydrate Countdown plan alone. This was a collaborative effort with many of my colleagues that took years to develop. First, myself and other dietitians at Stanford found that a diet was easy to follow if you were in a hospital and someone brought you a tray with just the right foods. But people don't live in a controlled environment like that. We live in a world where it's 2 P.M., you haven't had lunch, and the only available food choice appears to be the pizza being handed out at your son's soccer game.

"Second, we found that most diets are a bit depressing, because each bite of food is seen as a relentless drift toward fat. It's like thinking that when you spend money you're paying a fine. Most people don't think like this when it comes to money. Instead, they allocate a budget and use their resources accordingly. You can think of food the same way."

Tiffany had never thought of food like this before, but it made sense. There did seem to be a little pang of guilt every time she took a bite of food, but why? She needed to eat, didn't she?

"We learned that if people are given a budget of food each day—much like they have a budget of money to spend—they feel comfortable as long as they don't go into debt. Building on this idea, we were able to develop a strategy that helped people spend their budget as they pleased.

"In Carbohydrate Countdown, you eat, or *spend*, as you wish. No food is excluded. I won't try to fool you into thinking that some magical combination of food will miraculously reshape your body. Face it, the more you eat, the more weight you'll gain. But as you achieve your weight goals, I'll help you enjoy food and the role it plays in your life. In fact, I'll help you combine your food preferences into your lifestyle in a way that is pleasant, not depressing."

"And this will help keep me off diabetes meds?" Tiffany asked skeptically.

"It will definitely help. If you follow this diet, you'll lose weight, which should go a long way toward controlling your blood sugar. But are you ready for some even better news?"

Of course, Tiffany said yes.

"The beauty of this approach is that the very process of eating healthy and exercising helps control diabetes *even before you start losing weight.* You should expect to see better blood sugar control before you shed a single pound! I'll also show you some other lifestyle modification measures, including exercise, which will further help keep your blood sugar under control.

"So just as a sound financial budget leads to financial success, a healthy living plan, including your food budget, will lead to a successful lifestyle and control of diabetes. Happily, your lifestyle modifications will lead to an improved life in uncountable ways."

Whoa! A Budget?

Joanne could tell that something was bothering Tiffany.

"Tiffany, you look puzzled. Am I going too quickly for you?"

'No. But you mentioned budget. That isn't my strongest point. That's making me a little nervous," Tiffany replied.

"I understand," said Joanne, who in fact had been poring over her own financial accounts just before her appointment with Tiffany.

"I have some good news. A diet budget is not only much simpler than your personal finances, it is also easier to follow than the counting and worrying you've probably experienced before with other diets. You'll learn all about that when we begin planning.

"But more important to recognize now is that in this plan, you focus your attention on your single most important craving—carbohydrates. You don't even need to think about calories. They are in the background, of course, but you don't need to concern yourself with calorie numbers, anymore than you need to concern yourself with the nation's money supply when you write a check for your rent or mortgage payment."

Tiffany breathed a slight sigh of relief. But she still didn't feel that they were out of the woods just yet.

"In Carbohydrate Countdown, what you receive each and every day is a budget. How you spend it is your choice. Yes, you will eat some fats and proteins. Later, we'll give you a few simple guidelines for these items, but they will *not* be part of your budget. They are mad money, just like the $50 rebate check you forgot was coming in the mail."

Tiffany liked what she heard about the rebate check. In fact, it reminded her that she had a check coming for a microwave she bought a few months back. That brought a smile to her face. And the plan that Joanne was advising was sounding better and better the more she heard. Admittedly, she still had some unanswered questions and a lot of what she felt were valid concerns. But she was getting impatient. She was ready to get going.

CHAPTER THREE

The First Step

or, Can I please have my diet already?

O K, I'm convinced. Or at least this is worth a try," an exasperated Tiffany said. "Please give me my diet."

"We're getting there," said Joanne, trying not to acknowledge Tiffany's pained expression. "Remember, this is *your* healthy eating plan. In order for me to tailor your program to your own life, I have to know a few things about your life, your activities, and your eating habits. Even more important, Tiffany: You need to understand yourself as well as possible."

Tiffany was definitely ready for the next step, so Joanne asked her to keep a food record. "Write down everything you eat, when you eat, and how much."

"No way," she said. "I'm an administrative assistant. I don't need more paperwork in my life."

"But this is *your* paperwork," Joanne said. "You are doing this just for you, your own health, and your own happiness. Besides, I said this will be easy; I didn't say it would happen automatically. My clients who simply want to lose weight find they enjoy discovering new things about their lives. And those clients who have been diagnosed with diabetes have even more incentive. Just remember, Tiffany, that your success on this diet plan pays dividends in years of normal, vigorous good health—with the likelihood that if you achieve your goals, you will not need medication to control your diabetes."

Tiffany soon felt a little more reassured when Joanne handed her a very simple form to get started.

Take a break from Tiffany's story and look at
***Table 3-1. Workday/Weekday Eating Log* and**
***Table 3-2. Weekend Eating Log*. These logs are**
exactly like the ones Joanne gave to Tiffany. Use
these to fill out your own eating logs. This is your
first adventure in Carbohydrate Countdown. As we
follow Tiffany, you will have many more
opportunities to participate.

"It's very important," said Joanne, "to be as detailed as possible with this log. It's important not only to record every mouthful, but also to check off where you were when you ate. That can help us find patterns, and finding patterns is the best way to tailor the diet for you. On the sheet you'll see choices of *home, work, out,* or *on the go. Out* includes meals at restaurants or someone else's home. *Work* is any food you have during the workday. *On the go,* helps you remember to include those quick snacks in the car, at a sporting event, or strolling in the mall. Use these forms to record 3 days worth of eating and check back with me in one week. This is your first step in the Carbohydrate Countdown."

So Why Do I Continue to Gain Weight?

Tiffany arrived at her visit about a week later with a 3-day eating log—a weekday and 2 weekend days. Joanne noticed that Tiffany's diet, as she suspected, pretty much looked like it came from a guidebook for low-fat eating with few, if any, junk foods.

"Why the heck do I continue to gain weight," said Tiffany as Joanne perused the food record. "I think I gained

Table 3-1. Workday/Weekday Eating Log

Morning	home ☐	work ☐	out ☐	on the go ☐
Snack	home ☐	work ☐	out ☐	on the go ☐
Lunch	home ☐	work ☐	out ☐	on the go ☐
Snack	home ☐	work ☐	out ☐	on the go ☐
Evening	home ☐	work ☐	out ☐	on the go ☐
Snack	home ☐	work ☐	out ☐	on the go ☐

Table 3-2. Weekend Eating Log

Morning	home ☐	work ☐	out ☐	on the go ☐
Snack	home ☐	work ☐	out ☐	on the go ☐
Lunch	home ☐	work ☐	out ☐	on the go ☐
Snack	home ☐	work ☐	out ☐	on the go ☐
Evening	home ☐	work ☐	out ☐	on the go ☐
Snack	home ☐	work ☐	out ☐	on the go ☐

2 pounds this week. I guess it must have been the pizza at my kid's soccer awards banquet."

Sound familiar?

"Let's go through the record, Tiffany," Joanne said without further comment.

Check out *Table 3-3. Tiffany's 3-Day Eating Log* to see Tiffany's completed 3-day eating log.

Before going to the office, Tiffany ate a bowl of oatmeal, 1 large bagel, 2 cups of coffee with nonfat milk, and 1 teaspoon of sugar. This is typical for Tiffany.

At midmorning she began to feel a little lightheaded, so she had an 8-ounce glass of fresh apple juice and 4 graham crackers. She ate lunch at her desk—a turkey sandwich on wheat bread with light mayo, lettuce, tomato, fresh fruit, and tea with sugar.

About 3 o'clock, she walked across the street to buy a standard cup (about 12 ounces) of nonfat strawberry frozen yogurt.

Dinner included a bowl of vegetarian pasta with tomato sauce and just a sprinkle of Parmesan cheese. She accompanied the pasta with 2 slices of sourdough garlic bread and a green salad with nonfat dressing. Tiffany obviously was a fan of Italian food.

Notice how we divide the day into meals and snacks. Note that the "on the go" box is important. That's the place to mark that bag of pretzels you downed in the car on the way to pick up your daughter at daycare. Remember, you want to record everything, and we are going to try to make it as easy as possible for you to do that.

Table 3-3. Tiffany's 3-Day Eating Log

	Workday/Weekday			
Morning	home ☐	work ☑	out ☐	on the go ☐

Bowl of oatmeal
Large Bagel
Coffee with nonfat milk & sugar

| **Snack** | home ☐ | work ☑ | out ☐ | on the go ☐ |

Apple juice   8 ounces
Graham crackers   4 sq

| **Lunch** | home ☐ | work ☑ | out ☐ | on the go ☐ |

Sandwich with turkey, lettuce, tomato,
light mayo on wheat bread, Fresh fruit x 1
Tea with sugar

| **Snack** | home ☐ | work ☐ | out ☑ | on the go ☐ |

Frozen Yogurt   12 oz

| **Evening** | home ☑ | work ☐ | out ☐ | on the go ☐ |

Pasta with Tomato Sauce
1 1/2 cups Pasta   1/2 cup Sauce
Parmesan cheese, Garlic Bread   x 2
Green salad / dressing / nonfat

| **Snack** | home ☑ | work ☐ | out ☐ | on the go ☐ |

Tea with nonfat milk
Cookies   x 2

Table 3-3. Tiffany's 3-Day Eating Log (*Continued*)

		Weekend Saturday		
Morning	home ☑	work ☐	out ☐	on the go ☐
	1 Cup oatmeal Large Bagel Coffee with nonfat milk & sugar			
Snack	home ☑	work ☐	out ☐	on the go ☐
	Apple juice 1 Cup Graham crackers 4 sq			
Lunch	home ☐	work ☐	out ☑	on the go ☐
	Pizza 1 slice Diet Coke			
Snack	home ☐	work ☐	out ☐	on the go ☑
	Large Bagel Mocha Coffee with nonfat milk			
Evening	home ☐	work ☐	out ☐	on the go ☑
	1/2 Bag Fish Crackers			
Snack	home ☑	work ☐	out ☐	on the go ☐
	Tea with nonfat milk			

Table 3-3. Tiffany's 3-Day Eating Log (*Continued*)

	Weekend Sunday			
Morning	home ☑	work ☐	out ☐	on the go ☐
	2 Large Bagels with Peanut Butter Coffee with nonfat milk & sugar			
Snack	home ☑	work ☐	out ☐	on the go ☐
	Orange juice 1 Cup			
Lunch	home ☑	work ☐	out ☐	on the go ☐
	Turkey sandwich with lettuce, tomato, light mayo, on wheat bread Fresh fruit Tea with sugar			
Snack	home ☐	work ☐	out ☑	on the go ☐
	Berry Blitz Smoothie 12 oz			
Evening	home ☑	work ☐	out ☐	on the go ☐
	Pasta with Tomato Sauce 2 cups Green salad with dressing, nonfat			
Snack	home ☑	work ☐	out ☐	on the go ☐
	Tea with nonfat milk 2 oz 4 cookies, medium			

After paying bills and cleaning up around the house for a couple of hours, Tiffany drank a cup of tea with nonfat milk, and then she ate 2 supermarket chocolate chip cookies.

On the weekend, Tiffany ate a slice of pizza and a diet cola for lunch at her daughter's softball tournament, where the choices were limited. After the game, she quickly ate the bagel she'd left in her car. Then she stopped a half hour later when she found a branch of her favorite coffee house in a mini mall on her route home.

Rather than stopping for dinner, Tiffany and her daughter settled for eating the box of fish crackers they'd picked up at the mini mall. This was after each downed a 16-ounce mocha coffee made with skim milk. Stuffed with fish crackers, Tiffany drank some tea with nonfat milk before falling into bed, completely exhausted.

Sunday, she had 2 bagels with peanut butter for breakfast instead of oatmeal. For a midmorning snack, she drank a glass of orange juice. At lunch she had the familiar turkey sandwich she normally takes to work and enjoys making fresh on weekends. She also had her usual fresh fruit with tea and sugar.

Since it was Sunday, Tiffany decided not only that she had time to find a new blouse, but also that the trip to the mall would be the perfect opportunity for an afternoon snack. Tiffany stopped at her favorite juice bar for what the franchise called a 12-ounce Berry Blitz Smoothie. Dinner featured more vegetarian pasta, but she passed on the bread—the perfect excuse to eat 4 cookies instead of 2 for her bedtime snack.

Overall, sounds pretty sensible, doesn't it? Tiffany even budgeted in her cookies. So why does she continue to gain weight?

Joanne suspected there were some obvious and some not-so-obvious reasons. She asked Tiffany, "What did you learn from this?"

"Well, now that you ask, it seems I do okay except when I get sidetracked by my kids."

"Yes, Tiffany, your food choices seem to follow a pattern with regular eating times, except on the days when you're busy with your kids' activities. No one would criticize that. However, and you may not believe this immediately, you also tend to eat the same types of foods each day, and most of these foods are carbohydrates.

"I also noticed that on the weekend afternoon when you ate 'on the go,' you ate a particularly large amount of carbohydrates. By the way, that's why I asked you to check off *where* you ate. That helps us identify trouble spots."

"So what should I do?" Tiffany asked. She was ready for some answers. It had been three weeks, and she was still without a diet.

"Hold on," Joanne said. "We're almost ready for your budget. We're almost out of time today. I'll reveal the secrets to you at our next visit."

Tiffany let out an audible sigh.

Joanne continued, undaunted, "In the meantime, I've got an exercise that will help you understand a little more about how and what you eat. I'd like you to make an inventory. Please go through your kitchen and write down all of the food items in your refrigerator, pantry, and cupboard.

"Oh my gosh," Tiffany said. "That's a lot of work."

"It sounds like it, but it'll probably only take you about 20 minutes," Joanne said. "And you'll only have to do this once. If you feel confident, you can check the carbohydrate,

---

This is not an essential step. But as you'll see, the food inventory can be revealing and helpful. (And you might even find a few things so far beyond their shelf life that even your Aunt Mildred, who saves everything, would throw it out.)

Take a few minutes, like Tiffany, to fill out your kitchen inventory *(Table 3-4. Kitchen Inventory Sheet).*

Table 3-4. Kitchen Inventory Sheet

Food Item	Carbohydrate Group	Fat Group	Protein Group

protein, and fat column by each choice, or leave that task for later."

What *Is* a Carbohydrate? Or a Fat? Or a Protein?

Tiffany came back a few days later. She opened up a file folder with forms carefully filled out. But before Joanne could say anything, Tiffany quickly started.

"Okay, I've got a question. This word carbohydrate gets used all the time, but I'm not really sure exactly what a carbohydrate is. I understand potatoes, I understand bread, but other than that, what the heck *is* a carbohydrate!?"

Joanne sort of expected this. "Let's think of it this way, Tiffany. Of all the foods you eat, anything that originally grew out of or in the ground is a carbohydrate."

"That sounds simple enough," replied Tiffany.

Joanne continued. "Here's how it works. The sun provides energy, which is used by a plant's green leaves to put together water and carbon dioxide to form carbohydrate, which is often stored as starch in the roots of plants. That's what the plant lives on. Some of these roots are our most common foods—carrots and potatoes, for example. When you eat these foods, the carbohydrate is converted to glucose, and that's what provides energy to the cells in your body.

"Fortunately, or unfortunately, you don't have roots. Therefore, glucose is stored either in your blood to be used by your muscles, or in your liver to be released during exercise. If we eat more carbs than we need during about a 24-hour period, all of that excess energy can be stored as fat."

"So how does this affect my diabetes?" Tiffany wondered aloud.

"Well, I'm getting to that. The hormone insulin, which is produced in your body, directs the use and storage of blood glucose. Because you have type 2 diabetes, your blood sugar, called glucose, is stored and used somewhat differently.

Remember: A diagnosis of diabetes is made when the body fails to produce insulin (type 1), or when the body fails to effectively use the insulin it produces (type 2).

"It seems the insulin your body produces isn't doing its job.

"In either case, Tiffany, people who have type 1 or 2 face a similar problem: glucose builds up in their blood because there is nothing to tell the blood sugar where to go. Too much glucose can cause a variety of symptoms."

"I get it," said Tiffany. "As long as I stay away from roots, I'll be fine."

Joanne chuckled. "I think you know better than that, Tiffany. Carbs are everywhere. Besides roots, such as carrots and potatoes, we find carbs stored in many places throughout plants, including leaves and stalks. Certainly, green vegetables, and of course grains, such as wheat, rye, oats, barley . . ."

"Raisin bran?" Tiffany interjected.

"You got it," Joanne responded.

"How about fruits?" Tiffany asked.

"They are also carbohydrates, but they're a little different. They are fruit sugars, not starch. They are a simpler form of carbohydrate. But still, the bottom line is that fruit is used by your body for energy the same way as starch."

"So no matter what, all carbs are the same?"

"Well, Tiffany, not exactly. Some vegetables, especially greens such as collard, spinach, chard, or those stringy celery stalks, contain lots of water and fiber. Therefore, they have the least amount of carbohydrate. That's why you can eat more celery than bagels and not gain weight. But eventually, if your stomach could hold more celery, the effect would be the same as a bagel. Other forms of carbohydrate—dried beans, for example, the kind you make bean soup from—have much less water and are packed with carbs."

"Okay, I think I've got it," Tiffany responded, though the look on her face indicated she wasn't one hundred percent sure. "Carbs are anything that grows. If it doesn't grow, it's not a carb. Right?"

"There is one exception, Tiffany, and that's milk. Just remember that milk has to supply energy for little mammals, including human babies." Joanne paused before she finished the rest of her statement. She knew Tiffany wouldn't like what was coming next. "Of course that includes adult foods made from milk—foods like yogurt."

Tiffany went pale when she heard about yogurt. A life of bland celery stalks and boiled chard flashed before her eyes. A life without yogurt. A life without bagels. A life without triple mocha blends. She began to wonder if she could do this. However, before she panicked, she reminded herself that she was here to learn and that it was her health on the line. Besides, she was probably just over-exaggerating. It couldn't possibly be that bad (she would soon find that it wasn't). A little more collected, she took a deep breath and decided to get her mind back in the conversation. She thought a moment and interjected hopefully, "Cheese! That's a carb then, too."

Not wanting to shake her newly emerging confidence, Joanne thought this the perfect moment to introduce carbohydrate siblings—protein and fat.

"Well, the cheese-making process essentially extracts the protein and fat from the milk and 'wastes' most of the carbohydrate."

"Well, I do know that fat is really bad for you . . ."

"Not so fast, Tiffany," Joanne cautioned. "We need some fat because of the fat-soluble vitamins and other essential nutrients that it contains. If we ate no fat at all, our skin would dry and crack."

"I have enough fat stored on my hips to remind me that isn't my problem," Tiffany said with a sad grin.

"Let's not be too hard on ourselves," Joanne responded kindly. "Fats are useful because they add flavor, and they make us feel full and satiated before we eat way too much food. Fats, when eaten in limited quantities, can act as nature's appetite suppressant."

"Are all fats the same? Where should I look for fat? I'm guessing it's not only in donuts and whipped cream."

"Look for fats in meats," Joanne replied. "And we must also remember that fats are found in plant oils—for example, olive oil, and even safflower, corn, and the other similar oils. That's the part of the plant that isn't carbs—usually in the seed and nut of a plant, which is often the part that you wouldn't eat otherwise. And there is one exception to the plant carbohydrate rule—avocados contain fat."

Joanne saw that Tiffany was processing all of this information and while a little overwhelmed, she was proving to be a quick study. But they weren't out of the woods yet. They had one more issue to tackle—protein, essential for growth in younger years and repair of the body tissues throughout life.

"Your hair and nails wouldn't grow without protein," Joanne said. "Your skin wouldn't repair a cut."

"So where's the best place to get protein?"

"Eggs, meat, fish, poultry, milk, cheese, and yogurt are good. Vegetable sources are dried beans and peas, specifically soybeans and lentils."

"But I thought beans and lentils were carbs!!??" Tiffany asked, now a little frustrated.

Joanne took a deep breath.

"I wish it were that simple," the nutritionist explained. "But, Tiffany, foods can be made of a combination of carbohydrate and protein or fat, or for that matter, all three, or any combination of all three. We tend to categorize each food choice based on what it contains the most of. So you'll find dried beans and peas in the carbohydrate group, but while you're eating them, you're also getting the protein that you need."

"Sort of like a hidden food additive," Tiffany suggested.

"I guess you could look at it that way," said Joanne, enjoying the dialogue with her new client.

And Tiffany was anxious to move on. "Okay, Joanne, thanks for the lesson. I think it's all starting to make a little more sense. Can we take a look at my food record now?"

"Sure," replied Joanne.

The Eating Log Unchained

Joanne took Tiffany's eating log (*Table 3-4. Tiffany's Eating Log*) from the folder on her desk. One thing was certain.

"Tiffany, I'm going to give you the bottom line first. You eat too much. But don't worry. This program will help you with that and you won't even notice. Now, to begin with, let's break your carb intake down into CarboUnits."

"CarboWHATS?" Tiffany asked.

"In virtually all diet books and food labels, dietitians like myself and others typically divide food choices into 15 gram carbohydrate portions, sometimes called such-and-such exchange. For example, on cereal boxes, you'll often see 'starch exchanges' or 'carbohydrate exchanges.' That's basically what that is. Each one of these exchanges equals 15 grams. CarboUnits is just a term I happen to prefer, but the principle is the same; each 15 grams of carbohydrate equals 1 CarboUnit."

This is important, so it's worth repeating: **Each 15 grams of carbohydrate equals 1 CarboUnit.**

Joanne divided Tiffany's 395 grams by 15 to show her that she was averaging 26 CarboUnits each day (see *Table 3-5. Tiffany's Food Intake*). Tiffany was a little relieved you got to round off.

Table 3-5. Tiffany's Food Intake

In this table we converted all of Tiffany's food choices into grams of carbohydrate, based on food lists. Tiffany's total was an average of 395 grams for each of the 3 days. In fact, it ranged from 379 on her day at work to 417 grams on the Saturday she shuttled her daughter to the soccer game. Plus, we've taken it a step further. In addition to the raw numbers, we also divided this list into convenient CarboUnits, based on measurements that you'll find on a number of food lists and labels. **Each CarboUnit is worth 15 grams of carbohydrate.**

Time	Food Eaten	Amount	CarboUnits	Grams of Carbohydrate
Day One				
Morning	Oatmeal	1 cup cooked	2.0	30
	Bagel, large	1 = 4 ounces	4.0	60
	Coffee *with*	2 cups	0.0	0
	Nonfat milk *and*	2 ounces	0.2	3
	Sugar	1 teaspoon	0.3	4
		Sub-total	**6.5**	**97**
Mid-morning	Apple juice	8 ounces	2.0	30
	Graham crackers	4 squares	1.3	20
		Sub-total	**3.3**	**50**
Lunch	Sandwich:			
	Whole wheat bread	2 slices	2.0	30
	Turkey, lettuce, and Tomato with light mayonnaise		0.0	0
	Fresh fruit	1 medium	1.0	15
	Tea	1 cup	0.0	0
	Sugar	1 teaspoon	0.3	4
		Sub-total	**3.3**	**49**
Afternoon	Frozen yogurt	12 ounces	4.0	60

Time	Food Eaten	Amount	CarboUnits	Grams of Carbohydrate
Day One (*Continued***)**				
Evening	Pasta	1 1/2 cups	3.0	45
	Tomato sauce	1/2 cup	0.3	5
	Parmesan cheese	Sprinkle	0.0	0
	Garlic bread	2 slices	2.0	30
	Green salad	2 cups	0.6	10
	Nonfat dressing		0.0	0
		Sub-total	**5.9**	**90**
Bedtime	Tea	1 cup	0.0	0
	Nonfat milk	2 ounces	0.2	3
	Cookies	2 medium	2.0	30
		Sub-total	**2.2**	**33**
Total Carbohydrates			**25.2**	**379**
Day Two				
Morning	Oatmeal	1 cup	2.0	30
	Bagel, large	1 = 4 ounces	4.0	60
	Coffee *with*	2 cups	0.0	0
	Nonfat milk *and*	2 ounces	0.2	3
	Sugar	1 teaspoon	0.3	4
		Sub-total	**6.5**	**97**
Mid-morning	Apple juice	8 ounces	2.0	30
	Graham crackers	4 squares	1.3	20
		Sub-total	**3.3**	**50**
Lunch	Pizza	1 slice	2.0	30
	Diet cola	1 can	0.0	0
		Sub-total	**2.0**	**30**
Afternoon	Bagel, large	1 = 4 ounces	8.0	120
	Mocha with sugar	16 ounces	4.0	60
		Sub-total	**12.0**	**180**
Evening	Fish crackers	1/2 bag	3.8	57
Bedtime	Tea	1 cup	0.0	0
	Nonfat milk	2 ounces	0.2	3
		Sub-total	**0.2**	**3**
Total Carbohydrates			**27.8**	**417**

Time	Food Eaten	Amount	CarboUnits	Grams of Carbohydrate
Day Three				
Morning	Bagel, 2	2 = 8 ounces	8.0	120
	Peanut butter	2 tablespoons	0.0	0
	Coffee *with*	2 cups	0.0	0
	Nonfat milk *and*	2 ounces	0.2	3
	Sugar	1 teaspoon	0.3	4
		Sub-total	**8.5**	**127**
Mid-morning	Orange juice	1 cup	2.0	30
Lunch	Sandwich:			
	Whole wheat bread	2 slices	2.0	30
	Turkey, lettuce, and Tomato with light mayonnaise		0.0	0
	Fresh fruit	1 medium	1.0	15
	Tea	1 cup	0.0	0
	Sugar	1 teaspoon	0.3	4
		Sub-total	**3.3**	**49**
Afternoon	Berry Blitz Smoothie	12 ounces	4.0	60
Evening	Pasta	1.5 cups	3.0	45
	Tomato sauce	1/2 cup	0.3	5
	Green salad	2 cups	0.6	10
	Nonfat dressing		0.0	0
		Sub-total	**3.9**	**60**
Bedtime	Tea	1 cup	0.0	0
	Nonfat milk	2 ounces	0.2	3
	Cookies	4 medium	4.0	60
		Sub-total	**4.2**	**63**
Total carbohydrate			**25.9**	**389**

"So how many CarboUnits should I be eating?"

Joanne spoke softly. "About half the amount you're eating now. You should be enjoying 13.5 CarboUnits every day. I'll explain how I determined that in a minute."

"I still don't believe it. Where are all the carbohydrates coming from?" Tiffany asked. "It was the oatmeal, wasn't it?"

"No," Joanne said. "Let's go through your list.

"The oatmeal on Day 1 contributed 2 CarboUnits. But look at that giant bagel. You actually had the equivalent of 2 regular-size bagels totaling *4 CarboUnits*." Joanne pointed out that the bagels Tiff bought at the specialty bagel shop are twice as big as the "standard" bagels, so they provided twice the CarboUnits.

The nonfat milk and the sugar in her coffee contributed about half a CarboUnit.

Joanne looked at the midmorning snack.

"I guess it was the crackers," Tiffany asked remorsefully.

"Well," Joanne said, "the crackers contributed less than 1.5 CarboUnits, but the juice gave you 2 CarboUnits."

"Juice has that much?"

"Remember what I said about fruit. It's a carbohydrate just like bread and potatoes, just a different kind of carbohydrate. But a carbohydrate nonetheless," Joanne said.

Tiffany was ready for some good news.

"Your lunch was lighter," Joanne said. "The turkey sandwich, fruit, and sugar in your tea tallied just a shade over 3 CarboUnits.

There was really only one suspect left.

"It was the frozen yogurt, wasn't it?" Tiffany asked.

"Precisely. Your afternoon snack measured 4 CarboUnits, more than your entire lunch," Joanne pointed out.

Joanne could have sworn she saw a tear in Tiffany's eye.

"But I love my frozen yogurt," said Tiffany.

"Tiffany, if it's really important to you, no problem. We'll find a way to budget it in. They're your CarboUnits, you can spend them any way you want."

Tiffany looked relieved. Still, there was an evening meal and 2 more days left to look at. Joanne pointed out that the pasta provided a sensible 3 CarboUnits, and the tomato sauce and salad added a 4th. If she had stopped there, Tiffany would have totaled 4 CarboUnits for the meal. Not bad, if she had stopped there.

However, when she added the 2 slices of garlic bread, she added 2 more CarboUnits, and then another 2 at her bedtime snack with the cookies and tea. The bread and her bedtime snack cost as much as the pasta and salad.

"And you don't even get the pleasure of eating a nice, full meal," Joanne pointed out.

Continuing, Joanne went over some highlights of the next 2 days. Tiffany's breakfast and morning snack on day 2 were pretty reasonable, except maybe for the large bagel. But the afternoon was a disaster. Tiffany's afternoon snack reached *12 CarboUnits*, almost her entire day's budget, during a single binge in her car. It didn't get any better. The 1/2 bag of fish crackers added 4 CarboUnits. What Tiffany had thought of as a snack was actually packed with more CarboUnits than a typical evening meal. And Joanne had to ask Tiffany if the fish crackers offered the same variety and satisfaction as even the most ordinary evening meal. Tiffany just shook her head.

Fortunately, things got a little better. Day 3 was Tiffany's most sensible day, except for those 2 bagels at breakfast, which cost 8 CarboUnits. She was so close.

Tiffany thought for a moment. "Joanne, I think if I can keep my yogurt treat, I'll give up my bagels."

Bingo. Tiffany was well on her way to a successful Carbohydrate Countdown.

On to the Carbohydrate Countdown Ledger

Stuffed into the pile of papers in Tiffany's folder was her kitchen inventory, but Joanne told her to hang onto that. They were moving ahead.

"Later you'll see how knowing what you have in your house is a useful tool. But right now, let's get down to the real business."

Joanne handed Tiffany a pencil—with eraser—and her personal Carbohydrate Countdown Ledger, just like *Table 3-6*.

The ledgers Tiffany received from Joanne were pink, blue, and white. (Joanne thinks it's fun and motivating to copy the forms in various colors.) Tiffany liked the pink color best.

Tiffany noticed no foods were written in the blanks.

"This is your plan," Joanne said. "You will decide what goes in those spaces—with one exception. We will start with your daily budget written at the top."

Joanne wrote "13.5" in the space marked "Daily Carbohydrate Budget."

"You said you would explain to me how you came up with that figure," Tiffany said.

Table 3-6. Carbohydrate Countdown Ledger

Daily Total :	___ CarboUnits	(List Foods Here)
Morning	___ CarboUnits	
Noon	___ CarboUnits	
Afternoon Snack	___ CarboUnits	
Evening	___ CarboUnits	
Evening Snack	___ CarboUnits	
DAILY BALANCE	___	

"Because you're 5 foot 5. *We based your daily budget on one thing only—your height.* That's the key. Throughout your life you'll experience many changes. But whatever changes occur in your life, your 13.5 daily budget will remain the same."

"Okay. So what about the other stuff? CarboUnits can't be all there is to it," said Tiffany. "What about fats and proteins?"

"For now, you can ignore counting fats and proteins. We'll tackle those a little later. Let's start by focusing on carbs."

Tiffany looked a little apprehensive, but Joanne knew just how to put her at ease.

"Let's start spending your CarboUnits. You'll probably want to begin with your morning meal, which I recommend to be smaller than lunch or dinner. Eating a bit lighter at breakfast is often suggested for people with type 2 diabetes. That's because your body will handle food better if you start out slowly. Remember that besides your 3 meals, you get an afternoon and evening snack. Keep your goals in mind— optimize your blood glucose level and lose weight, too."

Tiffany looked at her food ledger and decided she didn't want to start with breakfast. First things first: she wanted to make sure she'd get her afternoon treat. So, she put a "1.5" in the blank marked afternoon snack. Joyfully in the space next to it, she wrote, "Yogurt treat." Then holding her breath, she looked up at Joanne.

"Well, Tiffany, it looks like you're going to have to make some concessions. If you want to get your frozen yogurt at the yogurt shop, it's going to have to be a very small cup to keep it at 1.5 CarboUnits. I think I may have a better idea. There is a yogurt treat that comes in tube packages, so you can eat them without a spoon. When you take them out of the freezer at home or work, they should seem just like a treat from the yogurt shop. Almost. You can eat 2 of these tubes at afternoon snack for your 1.5 CarboUnit treat."

Tiffany frowned slightly. "Well, it is yogurt," she conceded, "and it is frozen, and even better—I get 2 treats instead of one. And I suppose I could eat the tubes sitting on my favorite bench near the yogurt shop."

"Good," said Joanne. "Your balance is down to 12 CarboUnits. Let's continue the countdown with what you consider to be the most important food moment in your day."

Tiffany thought about the pressures of work, and how each day's lunch break was a welcome respite.

"My turkey sandwich and fresh fruit," said Tiffany fondly as she wrote those items on her ledger and in her mind deducted another 3 CarboUnits from her daily budget.

Tiffany smiled. "I still have another unit to spend at lunch. I think I'll have an eight-ounce carton of 1 percent milk. That will be good for my bones.

"Excellent." Joanne was pleased with how well Tiffany was catching on. "You have 8 CarboUnits left."

Tiffany put down her pencil, looked at her balance, and took a deep breath: breakfast, dinner, and one more snack remained. She decided to tackle breakfast first. She wrote in 2.5 CarboUnits to tally the oatmeal and coffee that she would enjoy with a half cup of 1 percent milk. Only 5.5 CarboUnits left to spend.

Tiffany began to see that her dinner budget, not to mention her evening snack, were going to require come creativity. Tiffany's pasta with shrimp and green salad totaled 3 CarboUnits. She added a gourmet touch—some kiwi fruit—for a total of 4.

"You're doing great," Joanne said. "Now you have 1.5 CarboUnits left for an evening snack."

"Well," said Tiffany, "my 2 cookies added up to 2 CarboUnits. I really do like the milk in my tea, so I guess it's time to make a choice. I think I'll just have one cookie, and I'll spend more time chewing it. There, I'm done." (Check out *Table 3-7. Tiffany's Completed Carb Ledger.*)

Tiffany took a quick look at her daily budget. She had been given 13.5 CarboUnits to spend, and she was pretty pleased with how she had spent them. Three full meals with room left over for an afternoon treat and a cookie to boot.

Table 3-7. Tiffany's Completed Carb Ledger

Daily Total :	13.5 CarboUnits		
Morning	2.5 CarboUnits	1 cup cooked Oatmeal	= 2.0
		1/2 cup lowfat (1%) milk	= 0.5
		coffee	
			2.5
Noon	4.0 CarboUnits	Sandwich with turkey,	
		2 slices bread	= 2.0
		lettuce, tomato, mayo	
		1 fresh fruit	= 1.0
		1 cup lowfat (1%) milk	= 1.0
			4.0
Afternoon Snack	1.5 CarboUnits	2 yogurt tube treats	= 1.5
Evening	4.0 CarboUnits	1 cup pasta with	= 2.0
		tomato sauce	= 1.0
		with shrimp	
		fresh fruit	= 1.0
			4.0
Evening Snack	1.5 CarboUnits	1 cookie	= 1.0
		1/2 cup lowfat (1%) milk	= 0.5
		Tea	
			1.5
		DAILY BALANCE	**13.5**

Building In Variety

Tiffany was about ready to leave (it was time to pick up her kids—and her afternoon treat), but Joanne had a pleasant surprise.

"Tiffany, this is an excellent start," Joanne said, "but it's important that we build in some variety right from the start. Here, take this. It will help you substitute foods and see what will fit into your budget."

Joanne gave Tiffany a Carbohydrate Countdown Catalog (see *Appendix A* for your own Carbohydrate Countdown Catalog).

"Tiffany, almost every carb you could think of eating is measured in CarboUnits. I've divided the list into logical groups that make substituting one item you like with something similar very easy. You can eat more of some foods than others, but if you stick to the Catalog, you'll stay in balance."

Tiffany looked at the list. It didn't have yak milk and a few other bizarre items that popped into her head, but Tiffany had to concede that the catalog did include virtually everything that she really was likely to eat. "So many choices. I'm afraid I'll get confused."

"I wouldn't worry about it. You'll build this into your life. And to make it easier, each of the portions in the catalog, with one exception, equals a single CarboUnit. The exception is Salad Vegetables, where 2 cups equal only 1/2 CarboUnit."

"That's almost like a 2-for-1 sale, isn't it?" Tiffany said wryly.

Joanne had another suggestion. "Mark some of your favorites with a highlighter. Notice we've put the choices in groups, so if you go out for breakfast, you'll find the pancakes listed right above the cereal choices in the same group—Cereals, Pancakes, Waffles."

"That's so easy," Tiffany said. "Maybe this isn't going to be so bad after all."

Joanne just smiled back.

CHAPTER FOUR

What About Me?

Tiffany went away from her first visit armed with a sensible daily budget and some options for making sure it stayed interesting and realistic. Now, you are ready to do the same. Let's show you the simple but unique way that Joanne determined Tiffany's budget of 13.5 CarboUnits per day, and let you in on some secrets that show you how figuring this is easier than you might imagine.

First, and foremost, your budget is based on your *height* and nothing else. Why? Because we've found that if you stick to the budget based on height, you'll reach your healthy, lean body weight naturally.

Lean body? We're kidding, right? The simple answer is no. To illustrate our point, try this basic exercise in front of a large mirror in the privacy of your bedroom:

Peel away the layers of clothing to that pair of shrinking underwear. Look into the mirror. *UGGGHHH!* No, it's okay. You're a grown-up. Get those negative thoughts out of your mind. Stay with us.

Next, stand with your feet about two inches apart. Relax with your arms at your sides. Breathe naturally and deeply, and adjust your body so you are equally balanced on both feet. Lift your head, look straight ahead, stand tall, and push your chest out slightly. At this point your shoulders naturally go back, your middle rises, your stomach moves in. Standing like that, tall and proud, close your eyes and imagine your lean body. You do have a lean body—it's just covered. Now turn slowly away from the mirror and walk tall. Feel lean as you begin this program.

Repeat this exercise each morning, midday, or evening to remind yourself that you are now eating for your lean body, not your old one. Keep that image throughout your waking hours. Think about it as you go to sleep. Then wake up and remind yourself of your leanness. The idea here is that you don't think of yourself as overweight. You now identify with your lean self and eat for your lean self.

Joanne had one client, Donna, who expressed this in a little different way, which worked well for her. Instead of focusing on self, she inverted the process and reached out to think of others. Donna, like Tiffany, had recently been diagnosed with type 2 diabetes and was feeling a bit sorry for herself. But one day it occurred to her that, "I can be healthy; I can be attractive. I am not going to let a medical diagnosis undermine my life. I will think about who I can become, not what I fear."

Donna observed lean women in restaurants and other eating environments and watched how they were eating. She observed what they ate and the speed at which they ate—much slower than her usual eating rate. When she ate lunch in a restaurant—which she often did by herself to relax and find a quiet moment on a busy day—she would think to

What Not to Do

While you are building your self-image, there is one tactic we *do not* recommend. *Don't make a daily trip to the scale.* We recommend that you weigh yourself no more than once a week. Your "weight" on the scale can fluctuate every day for a variety of reasons, including perspiration, hormonal influences, etc. This seeming rollercoaster can be disheartening and very misleading. Weighing yourself weekly, on the other hand, will help establish a trend over a period of a few months and will be a better gauge of your actual weight loss. Enjoy Carbohydrate Countdown. Don't become a slave to the scale.

herself, "What would the lean woman order, how would she eat?" By identifying with other lean women, Donna began to treat herself as a lean person. And eventually she *became* leaner.

Now, it's your turn. Look up your height on *Table 4-1. Daily Carbohydrate Budget At a Glance.* (No excuses! No fudging! If you aren't sure of your height, go measure yourself.) Then look to the center column to read your daily budget of CarboUnits.

It's that simple. Sure, if it were more complicated than that, we could probably sound more brilliant. But actually, we have put a lot of thought into this. You've probably heard it before, but often times the simplest design is the best design. For example, we found that our clients were able to stay focused and more successful when they directed their

Table 4-1. Daily Carbohydrate Budget at a Glance (for Women)

Height (feet & inches)	CarboUnits (15 grams/unit)	Total Carbohydrate (grams)
5'0"	11.0	165
5'1"	11.5	170
5'2"	12.0	180
5'3"	12.5	190
5'4"	13.0	195
5'5"	13.5	200
5'6"	14.0	210
5'7"	14.5	220
5'8"	15.0	225
5'9"	15.5	235
5'10"	16.5	245
5'11"	17.0	255
6'0"	17.5	260

attention to counting down carbohydrates, rather than tallying calories. Eating a planned budget of carbohydrates is your goal.

As we developed the plan, we were surprised at the simplicity. We kept looking for what else we might have to build in to make this work for almost anyone, things other than just carbohydrates and height. But the more we looked, the more we realized that was really all you needed to worry about in the beginning. As we move along, things like fat and protein will start to play a bigger role. Right now, all we need to do is help you peel away layers down to a leaner, muscular body.

To emphasize the mantra—Carbohydrate Countdown is designed to bring you into balance with your height. Your budget will remain the same when your lean body appears, and you get new underwear! You will be in balance, and your weight will remain stable.

So, find your budget on the chart, and take these simple steps:

- Copy several Carbohydrate Countdown Ledgers from page 40. (Indulge yourself. If you can, copy it in a favorite color or colors. Or color-code the copies— green for weekends and blue for weekdays, for example.)
- Write your daily budget at the top of all of your copies. This isn't going to change. Your budget has been spaced out through the day to make sure that your blood sugar levels are optimal. For weight control and general good health, the important number is the end of the day total, not each meal. But with type 2 diabetes, it's important to spend your budget wisely

through the day to make sure that your blood sugar levels are optimal.

- Plan your first 3 days. Here's how:
  - √ Look at Appendix B in the back of the book and find a sample daily menu that's been customized for *your* budget. If it makes you feel more comfortable, take items directly from the example to begin your first day of Carbohydrate Countdown.
  - √ As soon as possible, start substituting from the extensive Carbohydrate Catalog. Keep your life interesting.
  - √ Even if you follow our sample exactly, transfer the food choices to your own ledger. This will help you focus on your daily carbohydrate spending and help you maintain control of your carbohydrate budget. Take our word for it—keeping a ledger will help you stay on track.
- Start Carbohydrate Countdown *tomorrow morning*. Don't be too concerned with the amounts of other foods at first. We'll show you what to do with fats and proteins next.

And that's your first step. Before long, that leaner person underneath won't be buried anymore.

CHAPTER FIVE

Tiffany Comes Back for More

Tiffany's footsteps sounded lighter on Joanne's tile floor when she returned a week later. She told Joanne that she was really confident in her new budget planning.

"I'm feeling good about my carb planning, but I'm still a little unsure about fat and protein. Are these personalized for me, too?"

"No. We make it easy for you," Joanne said. "No matter how much carbohydrate is in your budget, your protein allowance remains the same—6 ounces of protein every day. All women need to include 6 ounces of protein every day."

"Is that *at least* 6 ounces? Can I have as much as I want?" Tiffany asked tentatively.

"No, just make sure to eat the 6 ounces every day."

Tiffany's head dropped. "Is this one more chore?"

"Measuring protein is really easy," Joanne explained. "And think of it as a bonus. It doesn't count as part of your carbohydrate budget. Look at the chart I gave to you (*Table 5-1. Protein Sources*). It's divided up into 1-, 2-, and 3-ounce sizes to help you divide the protein across the day. You don't absolutely have to spread the protein out across the day, but many of our clients say that when they divide their protein among breakfast, lunch, and dinner, they feel more satisfied and enjoy their daily Carbohydrate Countdown even more."

"Come to think of it," Tiffany said, "the day I substituted two slices of toast for the cup of cooked oatmeal, I put on

Table 5-1. Protein Sources

Eat approximately 6 ounces (oz.) protein daily from a variety of sources

1-ounce portion	2-ounce portion	3-ounce portion

Beef, Lamb, or Pork
1 oz. cooked meat
  (about 2 tablespoons)
	2 oz. cooked meat
	  (about 1/4 cup)
		3 oz. cooked meat
		  (about 1/3 cup or
		  1/4 pound raw)

Cheese
1 oz. cheese
1/4 cup cottage cheese
1/4 cup ricotta
1-inch cube hard cheese
3 tablespoons grated
  Parmesan
	2 oz. cheese
	1/2 cup cottage cheese
	1/2 cup ricotta
	2-inch cube hard cheese
	1/3 cup grated
	  Parmesan
		3 oz. cheese
		3/4 cup cottage cheese
		3/4 cup ricotta
		3-inch cube hard cheese
		3/4 cup grated
		  Parmesan

Egg
1 medium-size egg
  or 2 egg whites
1/4 cup egg substitute
	1 medium-size egg
	  plus 3 egg whites
	1/2 cup egg substitute
		1 medium-size egg
		  plus 4 egg whites
		3/4 cup egg substitute

Fish
1/8 cup canned crab,
  tuna, or salmon
1 oz. cooked fish
  (about 2 tablespoons)
	1/4 cup canned crab,
	  tuna, or salmon
	2 oz. cooked fish
	  (about 1/4 cup)
		1/2 cup canned crab,
		  tuna, or salmon
		3 oz. cooked fish
		  (about 1/3 cup)

Peanut Butter
1-1/2 tablespoons
NOTE: Here we suggest only 1 oz. portions, as peanut butter is so high in fat.

Poultry
the "little leg" on a
  chicken wing
3 tablespoons canned
  chicken
	a chicken leg
	
	a chicken thigh
	
	1/3 cup canned chicken
		1/2 of a whole chicken
		  breast
		1/2 cup canned chicken

Tofu (Soy Bean Curd)* 1/4 cup Tempeh	1/2 cup Tempeh	3/4 cup Tempeh

*NOTE: Contains CarboUnits: 1/4 cup = 0.5 CarboUnit; 1/2 cup = 1 CarboUnit;
3/4 cup = 1.5 CarboUnit.

a layer of peanut butter. That day I felt full right up until lunchtime."

"This list will help you not only choose protein selections, but also divide them," Joanne explained. "For maximum potential benefits, use 1 ounce at breakfast, 2 ounces at lunch, and 3 ounces at dinner."

"Can I substitute?"

"Of course. The choice is yours. For example, if you have a restaurant business lunch with a 3-ounce portion of chicken, plan on a 2-ounce protein portion at dinner," Joanne said, noting that Tiffany frequently didn't have meat at all at dinner.

"Meat at dinner," Tiffany said a bit wistfully. "You know, I think I should do that more often." Still, Tiffany looked a bit puzzled. "How do I measure my protein?"

Joanne was ready. "The surest way is to put it on a little kitchen scale. But you can estimate very easily. If you're cooking, you start with a 4-ounce portion from the butcher. Cooking removes roughly 1 ounce of weight per individual portion of meat. If you are eating cooked meat, 3 ounces is about the size of a deck of cards, or a large mayonnaise lid. You can also use a chicken to demonstrate ounces—a breast is 3 ounces, a leg is 2 ounces, and the meat on a chicken wing is 1 ounce."

Joanne and Tiffany went through the list together, noting that 1 egg is an ounce. Most sliced packaged cheeses are 1 ounce apiece, but you have to check the label.

Next, Joanne and Tiffany turned to the ledger for the happy task of adding protein. Tiffany saw that she was already eating her protein choice on days she had turkey at lunch. Her deli-size portion was about 2 ounces. Joanne explained how she could substitute another meat—roast beef, chicken, or ham.

"The fat content of lunch meat is about the same, so you can pick 2 ounces of whatever meat you like," Joanne explained. "Another choice is to cut back to 1 ounce of turkey and add a slice of cheese."

Tiffany liked that last idea, thinking of the Swiss cheese slices sitting at home in her fridge. Tiffany also liked the idea that she would be able to guarantee herself a meat, cheese, or similar treat at dinner. Better than a treat, she would be able to eat a full 3-ounce portion.

"I'm really looking forward to seeing that chicken sitting on my pasta," Tiffany said.

"And for variety and an extra health benefit, include broiled or baked fish," Joanne suggested. "Fish, especially deep cold water fish, such as salmon and tuna, have fatty acids that benefit cardiovascular or heart health."

"My husband has high cholesterol," said Tiffany. "Is fish something that would be healthy for him as well?"

"Yes," Joanne responded with enthusiasm, for she recognized that this meant Tiffany was understanding eating both for pleasure and health.

Breakfast was pretty easy. "What can I have?" Tiffany asked expectantly.

Joanne was ready again. "You get a 1-ounce portion of protein—an egg, for example. But remember how you felt better the day you had peanut butter for breakfast? You were energized all the way to lunch. A 1-ounce portion is 1-1/2 tablespoons of peanut butter. That should cover two pieces of toast nicely."

"That's true, the peanut butter did give me a bit of a pick-me-up. Why is that?"

"Because the peanut butter also contains some satisfying fat," Joanne explained. "It's one of those rare protein foods that naturally contains so much fat that we suggest you not use more than an ounce as part of your daily 6-ounce protein allowance."

"Speaking of fats," Tiffany paused. "What do we do about them? How do I work those into my diet?"

"You can add a visible portion of fat to what you're eating already."

"What's a 'visible' fat?" Tiffany asked.

"A visible fat is usually something you add to your food, like butter, oil, or salad dressing," Joanne explained. "It's not hiding in the food itself. I suggest a visible spoonful of fat with each of your three meals, using a big spoon and a small spoon. The smaller spoon, a teaspoon, is the size you use to stir your sugar into your tea. I suggest you use the small spoon for oil and butter. Then you will use a larger spoon, the size of a soup spoon, for salad dressings."

"But I've got a bigger question. What counts as a fat and how do I work it into my plan?" Tiffany asked.

Joanne spelled out a few fats that Tiffany could include. "A small spoonful of butter or margarine to go with your toast or sandwich. The small spoonful of vegetable oil you enjoy in your cooking—olive, canola, corn, safflower, or similar—can be your visible portion. Your salad can include a soup spoonful of salad dressing, or to make the salad more moist, mix some oil with vinegar."

"But if I have stir fry and have used my visible fat, what can I put on my salad?" Tiffany asked.

Joanne suggested flavored vinegar or fresh lemon to dress her salad. Tiffany was starting to like this eating plan even more.

For variety, Joanne suggested a soup spoonful of avocado, nuts, or chopped olives as visible fat. Tiffany thought this news was even better.

How about you? Are you ready to put your proteins and fats on your own ledger? Feel free to take suggestions from Tiffany's day and from the sample Carbohydrate Countdown menus in the book.

You can increase variety by borrowing menu choices from other height lists. For example, the lunch suggestions for persons who are 5 foot through 5 foot 4 are different. But each totals 3.5 CarboUnits. So, for example, if you are 5 foot 1, you can select the lunch choices from any of the other 3.5 CarboUnit lunch menu choices.

Table 5-2. Overview of CarboUnits in each Menu Pattern:

This handy chart will help you accomplish two goals. First, it will help you borrow menu choices from other lists. Just make sure that the number of CarboUnits for the meal or snack you choose is the same as for your height. Also, by spacing out your CarboUnits at 5 delicious stops throughout the day, you are helping to control your glucose, and thus, you are helping to manage your diabetes.

			Meal			
Height	Bkfst	Lunch	Snack	Dinner	Snack	Total
5′	2.0	3.5	1.0	3.5	1.0	11.0
5′1″	2.0	3.5	1.0	4.0	1.0	11.5
5′2″	2.0	3.5	1.5	4.0	1.0	12.0
5′3″	2.5	3.5	1.5	4.0	1.0	12.5
5′4″	2.5	3.5	1.5	4.0	1.5	13.0
5′5″	2.5	4.0	1.5	4.0	1.5	13.5
5′6″	3.0	4.0	1.5	4.0	1.5	14.0
5′7″	3.0	4.0	2.0	4.0	1.5	14.5
5′8″	3.0	4.0	2.0	4.0	2.0	15.0
5′9″	3.0	4.0	2.5	4.0	2.0	15.5
5′10″	3.0	4.0	2.5	4.0	3.0	16.5

Tiffany returns to her pantry and refrigerator

"Tiffany, you're really starting to understand Carbohydrate Countdown," Joanne said enthusiastically. "But before you leave, let's take a look at your kitchen inventory and see what you have in your pantry and refrigerator. This exercise should help you fine-tune your selections and make your healthy lifestyle plan progress even more smoothly."

Joanne had copied the list of food items in Tiffany's pantry onto a worksheet like the one on page 29. She asked Tiffany to go through the list and check whether each item was primarily a carbohydrate, fat, or protein. Joanne explained that a couple of the items belonged to more than one group.

Before you look at Tiffany's answers (which, for purposes of this book, are all correct!), take a look at your own inventory. You can use the blank version of Tiffany's list—we'll bet it has many of the same items you have in your kitchen. Then, as we go through Tiffany's list, see how similar it is to your own.

Table 5-3. Tiffany's Kitchen Inventory Sheet

Food Item	Carbohydrate Group	Fat Group	Protein Group
Beans, canned	✔		
Butter		✔	
Breads	✔		
Cereal bars	✔		
Cereal, cold	✔		
Cereal, hot	✔		
Cheese		✔	✔
Chicken breasts		✔	✔
Cookies	✔		
Corn chips	✔		
Corn, canned	✔		
Crackers	✔		
Cranberry sauce	✔		
Frozen dinner	✔	✔	✔
Fruit, canned	✔		
Granola mix	✔		

Table 5-3. Tiffany's Kitchen Inventory Sheet (*Continued*)

Food Item	Carbohydrate Group	Fat Group	Protein Group
Green beans, canned	✔		
Ground beef		✔	✔
Juice, fruit	✔		
Mayonnaise		✔	
Milk, whole	✔	✔	✔
Milk, skim	✔		✔
Noodles	✔		
Nuts, all varieties		✔	
Oils, i.e., olive, canola		✔	
Olives, canned		✔	
Pasta	✔		
Peanut butter		✔	✔
Peas, canned	✔		
Pizza, frozen	✔	✔	✔
Potato chips	✔		
Potatoes, instant	✔		
Pretzels	✔		
Refried beans	✔		
Rice	✔		
Salad dressing		✔	
Salmon, canned		✔	✔
Sodas	✔		
Soup, canned with noodles	✔		
Tomatoes, canned	✔		
Tortillas	✔		
Tuna, canned		✔	✔

Tiffany stared at her kitchen inventory for a moment. She realized immediately that most of her checks were in the carbohydrate column.

How about you?

"The potato chips! They were—are—for my kids . . . mostly. And they're *low fat*. They're baked." Tiffany sounded guilty. So Joanne reassured her.

"You have a pretty healthy pantry," Joanne said. "The main thing is to realize just how important those carbs are in your life."

Joanne continued with some important points. "Tiffany, here's the good news. This list is you. If you understand the items and can work with them, you'll be 90 percent of the way toward effortlessly counting CarboUnits."

"Just from this list?"

"Yes, because your eating patterns are fairly consistent."

And we are willing to bet that the same is true for you. I think we can safely assume that your food choices consist of about 50 items that you rotate through your life.

On Tiffany's list, there were 42 items, and all but 11 were carbohydrates—nearly 75 percent carbohydrates.

"You're surrounded by carbohydrates, which are really good foods, good energy sources," Joanne said. "But you're getting way too much of them."

Tiffany was a bit surprised to notice that there were more fats and proteins than carbs in her refrigerator. (Tiffany didn't bother to categorize the 1 pound of squid fish bait her husband had been keeping in the freezer for more than a year.) However, many of the fats and proteins also needed check marks in the carbs column.

"Milk," Joanne reminded her, "is a good example of a food that falls into two or three categories. The whole milk (which Tiffany said she kept for her kids) contains fat, carbs, and protein. Even skim milk is both protein and carbs. Cheese is primarily protein and fat. Peanut butter is both fat and protein."

Joanne pointed out that many of Tiffany's mealtime portions of visible fat are in her refrigerator—salad dressing, butter, and mayonnaise, for example.

And in her freezer were some of Tiffany's most prominent protein staples—ground beef and chicken breasts. She also had some frozen dinners, including a pizza, which also fit into all of the categories.

Tiffany frowned. "I'm starting to understand carbs, proteins, and fats. But this business about some foods being in more than one category is a little more than I can handle."

Joanne was expecting this.

"Right now, stick to the basics," she told Tiffany.

You may also be scratching your head a little. For you, the next chapter should help you sort out the ambiguities of combination foods. Fortunately, we have a secret weapon. You'll see . . .

Tiffany felt better. She had the basics to get her through the week, and the confidence that her remaining questions would be answered. She also anticipated unraveling the mysteries of a "secret weapon" Joanne had mentioned.

CHAPTER SIX

From Enlightenment Comes Success

Joanne noticed Tiffany's obvious glee when she returned a week later.

"I got it," Tiffany said. She told Joanne that not only was she becoming fluent in counting her carbs, but that the budget system really supported that feeling of control and well-being.

"Yes, sometimes I do feel a little bit hungry between meals and snacks," Tiffany confided. "But it really helps to know what I have to look forward to. In the early afternoon I know I have something sweet coming, and for dinner I can expect 4 CarboUnits. Then before bedtime I have another 1.5 CarboUnits to look forward to."

Joanne remembered that Tiffany had to modify her yogurt treat. "How did it go with the new gourmet yogurt treat?"

"Well, I have to admit that the first day I felt a little sorry for myself," said Tiffany. "But it got better. I decided I was really going to enjoy my afternoon treat—and the adventure of trying new delights. Instead of shoving large spoonfuls into my mouth as I walked back to my car, I made up my mind to savor my yogurt. I sat down outside the boutique and took slow, sensual, dainty bites."

Joanne saw success in every word.

Tiffany noted that reality sunk in a bit the second day. She was late to pick up her son from Tae Kwon Do class, so she had to eat a bit faster. "But I concentrated on that trail mix— all one-and-a-half delicious CarboUnits. I even reached into the bag and took out each piece separately, wondering each time whether I'd get a nut, a raisin, whatever. I know it sounds hokey, but I created my own sense of mystery."

Tiffany handed her week's ledger to Joanne.

"I'm really pleased with this," said Joanne. "It looks like you are adding variety to your day by making easy substitutions from the catalog."

For example, on Tuesday, Tiffany substituted an English muffin for her breakfast bagel. It was easy because a whole English muffin equals 2.0 CarboUnits, the same as half of her regular-size bagel. One day at lunch, she made her sandwich with pita bread, replacing the sliced whole-wheat bread.

"I really felt like I was getting an extra treat, because even though the whole pita was the same 2 CarboUnits as the 2 slices of bread, I was able to stuff in more raw veggies. I felt like lunch was a bit bigger."

The ledger also revealed that Tiffany had learned to substitute, keeping a close eye on the quantity. She didn't fall into the trap that somehow 2 *pitas* would equal 2 *slices* of bread. She didn't need that extra pita, anyway. She really enjoyed her lunch. But not everything was hunky-dory— there was a bit of overcast in an otherwise lovely week.

"I never realized how much pasta I eat," said Tiffany. "The first night I used all 4 of my CarboUnits for pasta. The 2 cups didn't fill my plate. I realize now that I'm used to eating at least twice that much."

Tiffany discovered that when she substituted 2 cups of mashed potatoes for 4 CarboUnits of pasta, she felt as if she were getting more food—the fluffy mashed potatoes just seemed to fill the plate a bit better than the pasta. She also discovered that rice might not be the best choice, since one cup of rice would cost her 3 CarboUnits.

"I will use my rice in a stir-fry meal, because then I'll have lots of vegetables to fill my plate."

"You're on your way," said Joanne, who was quietly working out a strategy to bring pasta back to Tiffany's diet. "Since pasta won't fill your plate, how about using a bowl.

One CarboUnit of pasta in a bowl looks much more generous than a 1/2 cup on a plate."

"That's a good idea," Tiffany responded. "I guess I never
thought about how important the mental aspect of eating
can be."

Wielding the Secret Weapon

Joanne guessed that Tiffany might have some questions. But
when Tiffany laid a veggie burger food package face-up on
the table, Joanne thought her mysterious secret weapon had
already been discovered.

"Looks like you've discovered the secret weapon on your
own."

Tiffany looked confused. "You mean veggie burgers?"

"No, Tiffany, not the veggie burger itself, but the
Nutrition Facts label on the back. Turn the package over,
and let's take a look."

"Great. That's why I brought it in. I thought this might
be a nice choice, but it's not in the catalog and I didn't know
how to compare it to anything else. Besides, it contains protein and fat, and I don't know how to deal with that."

"It's not too difficult," Joanne said. "Let's turn to the
label."

Joanne reminded Tiffany to look at the top to determine
the serving size, which is based on a typical portion. For the
veggie burger, the portion size was a single patty.

Tiffany noticed that the patty contained 1 gram of fat
and 5 grams of protein.

"The small amount of fat wouldn't even count as a visible portion of fat for this meal," said Joanne. "The protein,
5 grams, comes close to 1 ounce. Remember you need
6 ounces of protein every day."

Good to know—7 grams of protein equals an ounce.

Graphic 6-1. Sample Food Label

Serving sizes are consistent across product lines, stated in both household and metric measures, and reflect the amounts people actually eat.

The list of nutrients covers those most important to the health of today's consumers, most of whom need to worry about getting too much of certain items (fat, for example), rather than too few vitamins or minerals, as in the past.

The label tells the number of calories per gram of fat, carbohydrates, and protein.

Nutrition Facts

Serving Size ½ cup (114g)
Servings Per Container 4

Amount Per Serving

Calories 90   Calories from Fat 30

% Daily Value*

Total Fat 3g	**5%**
Saturated Fat 0g	**0%**
Cholesterol 0mg	**0%**
Sodium 300mg	**13%**
Total Carbohydrate 13g	**4%**
Dietary Fiber 3g	**12%**
Sugars 3g	
Protein 3g	

Vitamin A	80%	• Vitamin C	60%
Calcium	4%	• Iron	4%

* Percent Daily Values are based on a 2,000 calorie diet. Your daily values may be higher or lower depending on your calorie needs:

		Calories	2,000	2,500
Total Fat	Less than		65g	80g
Sat Fat	Less than		20g	25g
Cholesterol	Less than		300mg	300mg
Sodium	Less than		2,400mg	2,400mg
Total Carbohydrate			300g	375g
Fiber			25g	30g

Calories per gram:
Fat 9   •   Carbohydrates 4   •   Protein 4

Source: Food and Drug Administration 1992

Calories from fat are shown on the label to help consumers meet dietary guidelines that recommend people get no more than 30 percent of their calories from fat.

% Daily Value shows how a food fits into the overall daily diet.

Some Daily Values are maximums, as with fat (65 grams or less); others are minimums, as with carbohydrates (300 grams or more). The daily values on the label are based on a daily diet of 2,000 and 2,500 calories. Individuals should adjust the values to fit their own calorie intake.

Joanne reminded Tiffany that maybe a piece of cheese for another ounce of protein might be just what she needed to liven up the veggie burger.

"And to complete the visible fat with this meal, you can even have a spoonful of mayonnaise," Joanne added helpfully.

The veggie burger started to sound more exciting, but there was one more thing to deal with. Tiffany looked at the carbs. At 26 grams, her patty was almost 2 CarboUnits. (Remember there are 15 grams per CarboUnit).

Despite the picture on the wrapper, the bun wasn't included in the total Carbs for her patty. The bun would add 2 more CarboUnits, bringing Tiffany's lunch to her 4 budgeted CarboUnits. For somebody less creative, this might be the end of the story. But with visions of a veggie burger on her plate, Tiffany began to formulate options. There were several good ones.

"I really would like to have a glass of milk. That would add 1 CarboUnit," Tiffany noted. "How could I eliminate just 1 unit—eat half a bun and get my fingers sopping wet with mustard and ketchup? That's weird," said Tiffany.

Joanne had an idea. After placing her condiments and cheese on the burger, Tiffany could place a large piece of iceberg lettuce on the top to replace half of the bun, using the green to hold the ingredients in place. That way she could enjoy the bread and eat her meal like a burger.

"Well, that might look weird," said Tiffany. "But it might actually work."

Then Tiffany thought a moment. "How do I count one lettuce leaf?" she asked.

"You know you need two cups of lettuce to count a 1/2 CarboUnit, so one leaf of lettuce . . . let's just say it's free, it doesn't count as anything, " Joanne explained. "And you can even add some salsa to your creation without it costing you anything."

Tiffany suddenly felt sad. "Oh, gosh. I love chips, but I don't get any." At first her face dropped, but just a few seconds later, her frown was replaced with a smile.

"I could replace the bun altogether with 10 tortilla chips. 10 whole tortilla chips! I could layer the patty with the lettuce, tomato, cheese, and onions I would otherwise have put on the bun. Then I add some salsa, and voila—a taco salad."

From Little Cards Come Great Meals

Tiffany dug into her tote bag and extracted a pack of index cards. Joanne watched with interest. On 2 blank cards, Tiffany recorded in detail the pieces that made up her mealtime budget of 4 CarboUnits, listing the 2 variations she and Joanne had just discussed (*Boxes 6-1* and *6-2*).

Tiffany explained that she hoped to build a large collection of cards. Then, when she's ready to eat, she can find and quickly put together a good lunch. Joanne was very impressed. A little proud of herself, Tiffany said she had to leave and return the 6 overdue library books her husband had left in the car. Joanne, however, insisted that they needed to cover just a few more strategies using the secret weapon—the Nutrition Facts label.

Joanne brought out the box of a leading national brand of corn flakes. Tiffany quickly saw that the serving size was 1 cup. That was easy. She also saw there were 24 grams of carbohydrates. She instantly calculated this to be 1.5 CarboUnits.

Box 6-1. Card One	
Veggie burger patty.	2 CarboUnits
	1 ounce protein
1/2 bun	1 CarboUnit
Vegetables & salsa	FREE!
Mayo, one spoonful	1 visible fat
Cheese	1 ounce protein
8 ounces 1% milk	1 CarboUnit
Total	**4 CarboUnits**

Box 6-2. Card Two	
Veggie burger patty........................	2 CarboUnits
	1 ounce protein
10 tortilla chips............................	1 CarboUnit
Vegetables & salsa	FREE!
Mayo, one spoonful	1 visible fat
Cheese	1 ounce protein
8 ounces 1% milk.........................	1 CarboUnit
Total	**4 CarboUnits**

"You're doing this really quickly, but I can show you a shortcut. On this box, the CarboUnits themselves are already calculated and shown. These numbers were actually designed to help people with diabetes plan their meals. It will also help you with weight loss."

Tiffany was amazed. Joanne pointed to the bottom of the Nutrition Facts side panel. Printed in bold was the word "Exchange." Next to it was "1 1/2 Carbohydrates"—the same value as the CarboUnits Tiffany had calculated.

Like Tiffany, you should be aware of the carbs in your life. Pay attention to those Nutrition Facts labels. Learn to work with them by calculating the number of carbohydrate units in foods you commonly enjoy. The mantra is simple: "One CarboUnit equals 15 grams of carbohydrate."

Also, whenever you find a menu item that really works for you—like the veggie burger taco salad worked for Tiffany—be sure to write it down. But don't just put it on the back of a napkin. Put it on an index card—either paper or on your electronic organizer.

Joanne reminded Tiffany that CarboUnits were figured the same way as "exchanges" were figured for meal planning. This is the traditional measure of carbs, developed to help persons with diabetes. Sometimes the "carbohydrates" were called "starches" or "sugars," but the meaning was the same—one exchange equals 15 grams of carbohydrate, *or* 1 CarboUnit.

Alcohol in Moderation

One afternoon, Joanne heard Tiffany's voice speaking on her answering machine. "Please call me. I have a question," Tiffany pleaded.

Joanne was almost as curious as she was concerned when Tiffany came on the line that evening.

"Joanne, I went out for dinner and had a glass of wine. You didn't tell me how to count that!"

Box 6-3. Nutrition Facts: Shortcuts for Counting

Eventually, you'll be able to eyeball your portions with amazing accuracy, but until that time, here are a couple of helpful tools:

- *Scales and measuring spoons.* No, we don't mean that big scale you're tempted to stand on all too often. We mean a small kitchen scale for converting grams and ounces to CarboUnits. If it gives you confidence, by all means get yourself a set of measuring cups and spoons. To help identify a portion of visible fat, find yourself that small spoon from your cutlery drawer.
- *Your deli person!* Yes that friendly man or woman behind the counter will help give you portions down to the precise ounce—after all, careful measurement is how delis control inventory and stay in business. Your deli person will surely be happy to use butcher's paper or whatever to separately wrap your protein portions into convenient 2- and 3-ounce servings. You'll become adept at measuring those portions of sliced turkey, but to take out any doubt, your deli person can be your Countdown partner.

Joanne sort of chuckled. "Alcohol can be a bit of a mystery," she said reassuringly. "The truth is that alcohol is a bit of a wild card. Alcoholic beverages can contribute to weight gain, but except for beer or mixers, alcohol itself isn't a carbohydrate. Some experts believe alcohol is burned in the body more like a fat. Alcohol is kind of a special case."

"Yeah, okay. That's great," said an impatient Tiffany. "Now what do I do about it?"

Joanne explained that the single glass wasn't likely to be a deal breaker in Tiffany's program, although the definition of "glass" could make a big difference.

Tiffany interrupted. "What about for people with diabetes? Doesn't alcohol lower blood sugar?!" She was starting to get upset.

"Enjoy some alcohol if you like," said Joanne. " But it's important that you drink it with a meal. Moderate amounts of alcohol don't affect blood glucose *if* you drink that alcohol with food."

"What do you consider moderate?" asked Tiffany, realizing that was a key definition here.

"A good definition of moderate is one 5-ounce glass of wine, 12 ounces of beer, or a 1.5 fluid ounces of distilled spirits. Keep in mind that these measures may not be the same as what you or the bartender usually pour. To get an idea of size, pour a measured 5-ounce portion of wine into a glass. I think you'll find that 5 ounces is less than the usual glass you pour for yourself. Glasses in bars can either be more or less than 5 ounces, so it's important to gauge sizes or ask the bartender or wait person when you order. Keep in mind that soft drinks, juices, or any other mixes other than water are part of your budget and the CarboUnits they contain must be counted. For example, an 8-ounce glass of orange juice is 2 CarboUnits whether it's sipped at breakfast or as an ingredient in a screwdriver at a bar later in the day."

Tiffany mentioned that her husband says that alcohol burns calories before the body can use them. Joanne assured her that he was wrong.

"Remember, beer *does* contain carbs," Joanne contin-ued. "A 12-ounce bottle of beer counts as one CarboUnit. A 12-ounce light beer counts as 1/2 CarboUnit. If you drink beer, be sure to count it."

Tiffany had heard enough and came up with an idea:

"My life is complicated enough. I'm going to use wine as a relationship builder, not a drug. From now on, I'm going to have a glass of wine on weekends with Larry. Maybe some weekends I'll have two glasses. It will be a special treat for us," said Tiffany.

"That sounds like an excellent idea," Joanne said.

Your Good Friend, Fiber

The late night chat with Tiffany about alcohol reminded Joanne that there was something else they hadn't covered, something that Joanne was sure Tiffany would be excited about. Namely, winning the lottery. Well, at least the Carbohydrate Countdown lottery. While Tiffany had already begun to eat more dietary fiber, Joanne had a surprise.

"Your fiber is the carbohydrate equivalent of making a deposit," Joanne explained. Naturally, that got Tiffany's attention.

"It's almost like fiber is too good to be true," Joanne continued.

"Why is that?" Tiffany asked.

"Well, because this roughage in your diet acts like a bonus payment you can make to yourself. You've probably heard that fiber is good for you, but you may not know why. Let's just take a minute to describe it."

Joanne explained that fiber is the part of plants that we cannot digest. The message Joanne tried to get across was that fiber doesn't add CarboUnits to a diet, and it provides some great health advantages. Among the many benefits of fiber is that it improves regularity. And studies have shown that fiber may help prevent some common chronic diseases such as cancer or heart disease. Most public health guidelines currently recommend that all adults consume 25 to 30 grams of fiber every day.

"But for CarbCounters," Joanne added, "fiber is like putting money in the bank. Since your body doesn't use the fiber (it just travels right through), you can *carefully* deduct the fiber from the CarboUnit total of certain items."

"Deduct? How do I do that?" Tiffany asked.

"Like this. When, let's say, your cereal contains more than 5 grams of fiber in the serving that you eat, you get to subtract the fiber grams from the number of carbohydrate grams." Tiffany liked the sound of this. "For example, let's look at a cereal that provides 8 grams of fiber and 24 grams of carbohydrates (1.5 CarboUnits) in each 3/4-cup serving. Go ahead and subtract the 8 grams of fiber from the 24 grams of carbohydrate for a total carb count of 16. The happy news is that this reduces the number of CarboUnits from a little over 1.5 down to 1 CarboUnit. And keep in mind that the bulk in fiber will leave you feeling more full and satisfied than you would have felt without it."

"Wow!" Tiffany exclaimed. "But wait, does this mean I have to choke down those mystery drinks and bland cereals?"

"Not at all," Joanne reassured her. "Fruits, vegetables, and whole grains are all excellent sources of fiber. I can see from your eating logs, though, that you're like most carbovores—you avoid high fiber foods like the plague."

Tiffany looked a little sheepish.

"Well, don't worry, not a lot of people are attracted to things like brown rice, figs, kidney beans, or celery," Joanne continued. "Have you ever heard of a prisoner asking for brown rice and figs for their last meal?"

Tiffany laughed a little, but then a question popped into her head. "Can I have too much fiber?"

"It's hard to overdo, but yes. More than about 50 grams a day—remember that 20 to 35 is optimal—will probably result in stomach upset, and your body will have a hard time absorbing necessary minerals, such as zinc and calcium."

"Well," Tiffany confessed, "I don't think we have to worry about that."

CHAPTER SEVEN

Stay Alert!

Common traps and tips—Bargains, buyers, and social settings

I n this chapter, we'll take a break from Tiffany's journey through her Carbohydrate Countdown to discuss some common pitfalls of the healthy lifestyle. Just as your shopping life offers exciting special opportunities and potential bargains, so does your Carbohydrate Countdown budget. But beware! There are traps waiting to snare you as well. In the next few pages we cover some of the more common bargains and traps you're likely to encounter.

Traps and Tips

Sodium

Keep an eye on this stuff—it's the mother's milk of processed foods. We need a certain amount in our diet to stay healthy, but in our era, most of us get way too much sodium without even trying. It's everywhere. Sodium causes our bodies to retain fluid. Women during their menstrual periods are frequently vulnerable to this water-retaining effect of sodium. The answer here, of course, is to reduce processed foods and avoid putting extra salt on food. Spices, such as garlic, fresh herbs, cilantro, or parsley will keep food interesting without packing in the sodium.

Bulk

It may come as no surprise that the more you eat, the more full and satiated you may feel. This isn't always true, however. A pound of plain white rice probably won't have the same sense of fulfillment as a pound of truffles (we won't make any immediate judgments as to *what* the sense of fulfillment will feel like with either of these). But in general, more bulk is more filling. So take advantage of this scientific principle (or whatever it is).

The morning cereal selection is a good example of how this principle can be applied. CarboUnits aren't quite equal when it comes to breakfast cereal, because the density of various cereals is different. For example, several puffed cereals will let you have 1.5 cups for a single CarboUnit, while a popular wheat and barley cereal, Grapenuts, blows out 1.5 CarboUnits in a quarter of a cup. Part of this is ingredients; the other part is density. Puffed cereal has some air in it, so it doesn't pack quite as much density into each mouthful, but it's a mouthful nonetheless. The bottom line for you is that you get to chew more for the same dent in your food budget. Again, it's your choice, but for us that is usually a "no brainer."

Popcorn, as long as it has been popped with air instead of fat, is another example of a good munching food that is kind to your carbohydrate counting. By the same token, crackers usually aren't very kind. Many popular brands contain enough fat to make 5 or 6 crackers count as your visible fat selection for the day. (If you have any doubt that the fat is visible, look at the grease on your fingers after eating a few common crackers, or look at the grease spot the crackers leave if you put them on a paper napkin for a few minutes.)

Watch out for super giant economy sizes (and the stores that carry them)

These items, often sold at buyers' clubs or similar outlets, can give us the feeling that eating oversized portions is normal. There are also lots of budget-busting free food samples in these stores that can throw you off your plan before you buy a single humongous box of . . . whatever. When you do shop at one of these stores—let's face it, most of us think there are good values to be had—pass up the food samples unless you count the CarboUnits. When you come home with that giant box of cereal, immediately sit down and figure up how many portions and how many meals this box will cover for you and your family. You might even break the box up—divide the contents into CarboUnits and store each portion in separate plastic sandwich bags.

Giant soft drinks

These are even more common than oversized food portions. Fast food restaurants, ordinary supermarkets, and convenience stores typically sell drinks in humongous oversized containers under names such as "Big Swig," "Monster Mouthful," or whatever. They create a major minefield. If you must have a soft drink at the store, try a diet soda, which doesn't contain carbs and won't count on your budget. Keep in mind that diet soft drinks leave some people unfulfilled and psychologically ready to grab some food.

If you really want that coke with sugar, you'll need strong discipline, but here's a potential strategy: pour out 5 ounces—1 CarboUnit—into a cup you've brought with you to the store. Then throw the rest away or share it with a couple of friends. If it's a fountain drink, just pour 5 ounces into the smallest cup they have available. Remember to count the carbs, and tell yourself that the portion you throw away or leave unfilled is the healthiest part of this problematic snack.

Don't forget water

Water is a great substitute for diet soft drinks, and it's just a good idea anyway. About 8 8-ounce glasses of water every day is considered optimal. (Eight ounces is about the size of a paper coffee cup or a school-size individual milk carton.) If you work an 8-hour shift, you can drink one 8-ounce glass each hour of the work day. Designer bottled water is a fun way to "enjoy a drink" without blowing your carb budget. And do reach for water instead of juice, unless you really want to spend a CarboUnit or 2 on a snack. Hunger and thirst are different, but sometimes—especially when we're fatigued—it's easy to confuse the two. Don't let your body fool you.

Don't confuse the need for a nap for hunger

This is one of the pitfalls of travel. If you've flown by airplane, you've probably found yourself looking for a meal even though you've just had one on the plane (of course, airline meals are starting to become a thing of the past). No, you don't do this just because the airline meals are so tiny (if they're there at all). You're also responding to fatigue and possibly a shift in your body clock. If you're well rested, you're better in control of your body and you won't look for energy in all the wrong places. On the other hand, lying around the house all day pays no dividends either.

Expand your lists for variety

If you're a constant potato eater, don't forget to look to other sources of carbs with your meals—pasta, rice, bulgar, the list goes on. As a carbovore (or carboholic, or whatever term you prefer), you have the potential to be flexible with your choice of carbohydrate staples. Take advantage of your appetite to create variety in your meals. Plus, some forms of carbohydrates, including many pastas, are less dense and let you increase your portion size without taking a bigger bite out of your budget.

Remember that fat-free items can be an evil trap

Fat-free cookies, cakes, cheese, all manner of snack foods, and almost everything else have become ever-present in our society. They're everywhere. Even if you're on a low-fat diet, we don't recommend relying on these processed fat-free items. Check the carbohydrates. Usually, you're not saving much, if anything, on your budget, and you'll feel less satisfied and be tempted to eat more. Almost everybody who's tried them agrees that the cookies and crackers, for example, don't taste as good as their originals, so they leave you less satisfied.

We recommend that you budget in some "real" food, and swap the fat-free "fake" goodies for something that is naturally low in fat or fat-free. A carrot labeled fat-free is exactly the same as a carrot with no label, but you get the point.

If you're the family food preparer, watch out for some common pitfalls

The food you taste during preparation counts on the Carbohydrate Countdown plan. And so does baby food that you eat to show a little one how he or she is supposed to eat. Does your family really need to see you eat huge portions to believe the food you gave them is okay? We'll make an exception for the official royal taster in a beleaguered feudal monarchy, but for the other 99.9999% of you, try this phrase: "I made it, it's great, eat it or leave it."

Resist well-meaning but bad advice

Sometimes it's hard to ignore the well-meaning suggestions, or pressure, from your friends and family. Talk to your spouse if he or she tempts you to eat more and stray from Carbohydrate Countdown. Family members can sometimes be critical, and their advice isn't necessarily helpful or rational. Explain why you need to discipline yourself. Perhaps more important, let your family know they are not necessarily bad eaters because of what *they* consume. In fact, for the most part, everybody is sharing the same meal.

Be creative with portion size

Tiffany, for example, often cooks two vegetables for dinner instead of one. She enjoys some of each, and feels satisfied without going over her budget by eating too much pasta, potato, or bread. Yet, her plate is full. In fact, Tiffany's husband has complimented her on the variety of her meals. He likes a second vegetable, too. Now, Tiffany cooks even more so that she has some left over for lunch the next day.

Gifts

What did you do with all that candy the kids brought home at Halloween? What about the sweets you received from grateful clients, neighbors, or whomever for the holidays? One thing that's important: Don't leave that food out where you nibble on it! You might give it away to a senior or youth center where there are so many worthy recipients that no one person will have an opportunity to pig-out on all the candy.

Don't fixate on the scale!

We can't emphasize this enough. Remember to weigh yourself no more than once a week. Daily weighing is misleading—because it involves fluctuations unrelated to your budget—and it diverts your attention away from the pleasures of eating, causing you to focus on the fact that you are still a work in progress.

CHAPTER EIGHT

Movin'

Working exercise into an everyday routine

A few weeks later, Joanne asked Tiffany to complete an activity log, which is a good idea for you as well. A good exercise program is probably as important to your diet as your food choices. If that sounds daunting, don't even call it exercise. Call it movement. Put simply, you need to move, and how you do that is your choice.

You may wish to talk with your doctor about how diabetes might influence your exercise program. But chances are—as long as you are otherwise healthy—you will have to make few, if any, accommodations when it comes to keeping fit. In fact, the vast majority of people find that a solid exercise routine reduces symptoms and the effects of complications. If you're a highly active athlete who's just been diagnosed with diabetes, you do need to talk with your doctor and trainer. Extremely vigorous exercise may require some adaptive strategies to keep your blood glucose in check. But if you have no symptoms, don't use your diabetes as an excuse to avoid exercise. Even intense athletic training can be realistic and beneficial for those otherwise in good health.

Surprisingly, you may be doing a fair amount of moving already. That's why it's important to complete a one-week log to realistically find where you are now, and what you might need to do to make this part of your life more beneficial.

So, Tiffany completed her movement log (*Table 8-1. Tiffany's Movement Log*). We've also included a blank log for you (*Table 8-2. Blank Movement Log*).

We haven't listed specific activities, because the choice is yours. And the choices are infinite—from mowing the lawn and vacuuming the living room to climbing a 7-kilometer peak in the Himalayas. Every time you do one of these activities, write down the number of minutes you spend. Did you rake the leaves this weekend? Count the minutes. Did you park your car 15 minutes from the store when you went grocery shopping? Write down the time you spent walking to your destination—and back.

Recent studies have shown that exercise for health is beneficial in light, short intervals. Where people often become confused is that such light, sporadic exercise doesn't build athletic prowess. But it *will* help you expend carbs, and evidence is mounting that it provides multiple health advantages.

You may not want to record everything at the time you do it. For example, if you have a few minutes at work and want to climb up to the next floor, wait to record a few of these excursions when you have a few seconds at your desk to jot them down. Record what you're doing, and better yet, note what you'd *like* to be doing in the blanks on the left side of the page. That will remind you to try something new when you get time.

Tiffany's Active Lifestyle

Tiffany had a broad smile on her face when she returned with her filled-out log the following week. She was enjoying Carbohydrate Countdown, finding delicious substitutions that didn't tax her 13.5 CarboUnit budget. She hadn't weighed herself after Joanne told her, "develop the budget, the weight loss will come." (Remember, weighing yourself too often will only create needless apprehension.) But Tiffany knew she was successful—her jeans were fitting a bit better.

Table 8-1. Tiffany's Movement Log

Record time using 15-minute intervals; for example:
15 mins, 30 mins, 45 mins, or 1 hour.

Activity	Sun (mins)	Mon (mins)	Tues (mins)	Wed (mins)	Thurs (mins)	Fri (mins)	Sat (mins)
cleaning		45	15	15		30	
vacuuming							
OTHER	washing car 30						
snow shoveling							
raking leaves							
mowing lawn							
gardening	60						
walking							30
climbing stairs		15	15	15	15	15	
climbing/hiking							
using a treadmill							
biking							45
dancing							
rowing							
swimming							
playing tennis							
riding a stationary bike							
doing yoga				60			
skating							
golfing							
bowling							
Subtotal	90	60	30	90	15	45	75
WEEKLY TOTAL							**405 MINUTES**

Table 8-2. Blank Movement Log

**Record time using 15-minute intervals; for example:
15 mins, 30 mins, 45 mins, or 1 hour.**

Activity	Sun (mins)	Mon (mins)	Tues (mins)	Wed (mins)	Thurs (mins)	Fri (mins)	Sat (mins)
Subtotal							
WEEKLY TOTAL				_____ **MINUTES**			

Joanne looked at Tiffany's activity log. Sunday was Tiffany's most active day. Instead of suggesting that her husband, Tom, wash the car, Tiffany decided to take it to the car wash. But then she remembered her activity log and washed it herself, proudly recording 20 minutes. She had debated whether to vacuum the carpets and wash the inside of the car windows, but she convinced herself to do so when she recalled that these would add an extra 10 minutes to her log. When she finished, Tiffany stared lovingly at her sparkling clean Honda coupe. Then she stared lovingly at the large package of M&Ms she had moved to the front seat from the backseat while vacuuming. But her higher instincts prevailed when she read the nutrition label on the candy wrapper. "Two CarboUnits!" she almost shrieked. "No way. That's half my lunch budget." Tiffany put the candy back in her pocket, saving it for her daughter who would probably want a snack after soccer practice. Energized, Tiffany added another 60 minutes to her activity log by cleaning her flowerbeds and adding some primroses.

"You know, Joanne, a clean car and some freshly planted flowers was almost as rewarding as . . . well, as food."

"Feels good, doesn't it? You're off to a great start," Joanne said.

The rest of the week wasn't quite so active, with work and kids to shuttle. Since Tiffany spent most of her weekend outside, she put in a 45-minute burst of energy inside on Monday, cleaning those parts of the house visitors were likely to see. On Monday, Tiffany noted how much time she spent climbing the stairs to her 3rd floor office. The log encouraged her to avoid the elevator altogether (except once when her boss started talking to her as they were both going up to the 3rd floor). And a few times Tiffany found an excuse to add a trip, because she found it would bring her tally up to 15 minutes—her personal stair-climbing goal.

Tuesday, she fell back into her usual routine of putting in 15 minutes of housecleaning before getting ready for work. She cleaned a little bit faster than usual—she was feeling energized and wanted to make sure she really was "movin'."

She finished her regular cleaning 2 minutes earlier at the faster pace, so she spent the 2 bonus minutes picking up and taking her husband's old golfing magazines to the recycling bin.

Tiffany told Joanne that the housework was actually a bit easier, knowing she could put the time on her activity log.

On Wednesday, she went to her yoga class at the YMCA. This was not new. Tiffany had always looked forward to this respite from stress in the middle of her busy workweek, and it felt especially good to log an hour of exercise, as well as enjoy the spirit of the yoga.

Thursday, she had a major proposal to clean up for her boss, and so she didn't even get her 15 minutes of cleaning in the morning.

On Friday, though, she spent 30 minutes cleaning and vacuuming, spurred both by the need to add to her activity log and the impending visit the next day from her mother-in-law, Bernice.

On Saturday, Tiffany took a 30-minute walk with Bernice to her favorite coffee shop. Tiffany was able to find a 2.5 CarboUnit breakfast listed on the 5-foot-3 menu. She ordered oatmeal. The portion of oatmeal at Jumbo Sam's Coffee Emporium was bigger than the cup her menu plan called for, but Tiffany had a simple strategy. She sprinkled the budgeted spoonful of raisins on top, poured some low-fat milk on the surface, and began eating a cupful of oatmeal. Tiffany ate slowly and *did not eat the entire bowl of oatmeal*, instead stopping after about a cup. Because Tiffany had enjoyed her breakfast, Bernice didn't even know Tiffany was CarbCounting. After refusing Tiffany's offer to share the leftover oatmeal, Bernice did make a comment about wasting food, but she backed down when Tiffany offered to ask the waitress for a take-home container. (Tiffany knew that Sam, the proprietor, fed all leftovers to his St. Bernard, Ollie.)

Because Tiffany was really looking forward to lunch, she could comfortably refuse Bernice's offer of a bear claw on the way out from Sam's. And Tiffany felt in control, although a bit envious, while she watched Bernice eat *her* bear claw as they walked down the street.

In the afternoon, while Tom helped Bernice fill out her taxes, Tiffany's kids joined their mom on a 45-minute bike ride that included a stop at the video store to return a movie she and Tom had watched the night before. Originally, she had planned to drive to the video store. But then she remembered her activity log, and even though she had a lot planned that Saturday, she figured the little extra time it would take on her bike was well worth it because of the minutes it would add to her log. So she had her son, Kevin, plump the tires on her long-neglected 10-speed and the group pedaled away.

How much is enough?

After Tiffany had told Joanne about her week's activities, Tiffany popped the big question.

"Am I movin' enough? How much exercise should I be getting?

"Looking at the log, Tiffany, it seems that you added a couple of really good activities this week—the car wash and the bike ride. These seem to fit in very comfortably with your lifestyle. Do you think, overall, that this is as much activity as you would like to get?"

"I used to do more," Tiffany said a bit sadly. "In fact, I think of myself as an active person, but realized doing this log that a lot of that is based on what I used to do, or did occasionally."

"That's very normal," Joanne reassured her. "And that's one reason we do the log—to create a ledger of our activity, to get in touch with reality. That being said, I can now answer your question. You are basically healthy, so you can safely work in more exercise. And working in more exercise would benefit you quite a bit."

"But how can I do that?" Tiffany sounded stressed.

"You're already doing it," Joanne said. "The bike ride and car wash are good examples of that. The extra time it took to ride your bike, an outstanding activity, to the video store, was small. But wasn't it more fun to enjoy an activity with your kids than to argue with them sitting in the car?"

"Okay, more is good, but help me get some sense of how much I need," Tiffany said.

Joanne understood that Tiffany needed some specific direction.

"Let's plan this out. Most experts recommend that you need about 30 minutes of activity most days—though not necessarily in one time block—to maintain good health. But anything over that should make carb counting and the rest of your life more effective. When you add some vigorous exercise to your routine—a brisk bike ride, for example— you can expect to gain added fitness benefits, as well as health and weight loss perks. Right now, let's work from your baseline . . ."

"My what?" Tiffany asked, a little bit wary of this out-of-the-blue terminology.

"You're doing a certain level of exercise without even thinking of it as such; we'll call that your baseline. That includes the cleaning in the morning, climbing stairs at work, and your midweek yoga class. On weekends you're more than doubling your activity with a combination of chores and fun.

"We'll make it simple. Your first task is to make sure you don't drop below the 30-minute daily minimum on week-days, and the 90-minute combination of activities on week-ends. You've already got these pretty well plugged into your routine, so you can focus your attention on finding new things to enhance your life."

"When you put it that way," Tiffany said, "it sounds a little less daunting. In fact, it sounds good."

Tiffany looked as if she'd just thought of something. "Can I lose weight faster if I exercise longer?"

"Yes, Tiffany, you can. But let's be realistic. You have three alternatives, with variations, all of which are okay. First, if you really, truly feel that you can't afford any more time or effort, go ahead, continue with what you're doing. It's a baseline and carb counting will continue to work.

"Second, if you want to lose weight a bit faster, figure out how you can add 15 minutes during the week, and an extra half hour on each weekend day. For example, maybe you could take a 15 minute walk at lunch."

"I could do that," Tiffany said. "The weather is getting better, and I can leave an extra pair of walking shoes under my desk. Fifteen minutes isn't much. I could almost do that by walking up and down the corridor a few times."

Tiffany thought a moment. "Okay, what's alternative three?"

Joanne nodded. "I think you know," she said.

"Yes," Tiffany said, "it's back to the Y for a real aerobics program. I used to go 2 to 3 times a week before my kids' lives got more complicated than mine. Maybe I could start again. How much faster will carb counting work if I do that?"

"I wouldn't look at it that way. The answer is the more you do, the faster you'll lose weight, and in most cases, the better you'll feel. And statistically, you'll reduce the possibility that your type 2 diabetes will become more complicated. Exercise generally has been shown to reduce the risk factors for other chronic conditions, such as heart disease," said Joanne.

"Exercise, even at the more modest but realistic levels that you're achieving, brings real weight loss. It's not just a temporary drop that can occur if you periodically starve yourself. The weight loss is a bonus. Good health is the real advantage."

Tiffany thought for a moment. "I think I can get back to the gym twice a week. When I'm there, I can make it a point to be vigorous."

Joanne handed Tiffany a blank movement log and told Tiffany this time to fill it in with *planned* activities. Joanne also told her to put in her baseline activities, as well.

"Combining what you're doing with what you'd like to add on a weekly planning sheet will help you understand how to budget your time and fit in those extra moves."

Tiffany wrote down her baseline activities and paused.

"You know, I think realistically that if I add a lunchtime walk four times a week (leaving one day open for the inevitable staff meeting or trip home to pick up her kid for a dentist appointment), and keep my yoga class, I'll only get to the gym one other night during the week."

Joanne didn't say anything. Tiffany appeared to keep thinking.

"Come to think of it," Tiffany finally said. "Tom and I usually manage to get out for dinner one night a week. I'll bet I could convince him to take the ballroom dancing class that we've been kidding each other about."

Tiffany penciled in ballroom dancing for Friday night. It was time spent with her husband—but it would also count on her exercise log.

You can see how Tiffany began to put movement into her life. We hope you are doing the same at this point. Start with your movement log—you can look at Tiffany's to get some ideas. After you discover your baseline for a week, make a realistic appraisal of ways to add more. How much more? As we discovered with Tiffany, that's up to you, as long as you reach your baseline of 30 minutes of activity every day. The most important point is to add at least something to the baseline and try never to let your movement drop below your baseline of 30 minutes most days each week.

Box 8-1. Movement Checklist

✔ Do *something* every day for 30 minutes.

✔ Don't look at exercise as an add-on to your life. It must be part of your life.

✔ Look for ways to modify usual activities to incorporate movement. For example, use the stairs instead of the elevator.

✔ Combine activities. If you need to buy milk at the neighborhood market, walk or ride your bike instead of driving.

✔ Gradually increase what you do. For example, if your exercise consists of parking your car a few blocks from work and then walking in, start parking a few blocks even farther away. Gradually increase the distance until you start counting by miles instead of blocks.

✔ Try to select fun activities. A pleasant and relaxing walk by the river or in the woods 5 days a week, a walk you stick with, is far more beneficial than 30 minutes of vigorous running—if the running program is so unpleasant to you that you only get to it once a week.

✔ **Use your log sheet.** It will help you keep track of what you *really* did to move. And it will help keep you motivated—after all, you don't want a blank spot 3 days in a row, do you? You'll probably find the log sheet encouraging. Maybe on Thursday you didn't get to the gym, but you did park your car at the very end of the lot. This offered an opportunity for a brisk 1/4-mile walk to the office. Write it down. You earned it.

Tiffany's Neighbor Betty Gets Movin'—Without Fear

Tiffany's good friend, Betty, was able to turn an unpleasant situation into an opportunity for success. Betty's story may sound familiar. If so, maybe you can glean some inspiration from her tale of triumph.

When Tiffany walked to Betty's house to replace the camera batteries she had borrowed the week before, her neighbor sat in the kitchen looking despondent.

"I don't know what looks worse," said Betty, "the pile of clothes mounting on my exercise bike or me."

Tiffany understood the dilemma. Betty, a busy secretary who always liked to look good, had given up on working out at a gym because she said she was too embarrassed to have anyone see her in workout clothes. Betty wanted to exercise but was too self-conscious, even at home.

"Whenever I get on the bike, it seems as if Larry laughs and jokes. I know he isn't trying to be cruel, but whenever I take the clothes off the bike and get on to ride, he tells me, 'Looks like you replaced the pile of clothing with two laundry bags.'"

Tiffany didn't think that was very funny. "You can't let Larry's insensitivity stop you from doing the right thing for yourself," she said.

Tiffany and Betty talked, and they decided that until she climbed on that exercise bike, her hips and thighs weren't going to get any smaller. But she was also realistic and realized that even though she wished it wasn't so, she was going to have to work around her husband's quips and "harmless" insults. From that day forward, she got on the bike only when Larry wasn't watching, usually early in the morning before he got up. Pretty soon, her program became consistent and enjoyable.

After awhile, she felt confident enough to venture out to the YMCA, where she joined an exercise class of equally positive and confident women (and a few men, too). She may still have been a little large, but because her experience at home had made her comfortable with an exercise environment, she wasn't self-conscious and felt pleased that she was able to take some control of her life.

A few months after Betty began her routine, Tiffany came over to Betty's house to drop off the schedule for a local amateur theater. Betty was upstairs on the exercise bike. Yes, she continued to go to the gym, but on days when her class didn't meet, Betty liked to squeeze in an extra 20 minutes or so before she had to start cooking dinner—on those days when her husband didn't come home early to cook. Eventually, Betty found the confidence to seek counseling, and soon after, Larry agreed to join her. After some tough discussions, Larry began to understand Betty's viewpoint a little better, while a less frustrated Betty became a little easier to get along with.

Sound impossible? Well, we'll keep saying it, but it's true. Exercise can become the best "addiction" you'll ever find.

Remember, family members need to respect your need to exercise and have time of your own. Both of these fulfill important nutritional and psychological goals.

From ridicule to guilt

Unfortunately, Betty and her husband weren't through with their problems just yet. Even after Betty learned how to exercise away from her husband's critical eye, she found she once again had a barrier to cross.

Betty started the carbohydrate countdown and stuck with it for a year. Her exercise program thrived, and during the course of the year, she lost 15 pounds and was well on her way to an ideal weight only 5 pounds away.

Then she lost her job.

Instead of giving her free time, Betty, like many people in similar situations, found she was actually busier. For one thing, her 14-year-old son, Myron, had started taking computer classes at the local junior college, classes she had to take him to. She also found that looking for a hairdressing job (she was through being a secretary) that fit her personality, hours, and need for creativity could well use up more than 20 hours a week. After dinner, her husband Larry, picking up a stack of unpaid bills from the desk, would pointedly ask Betty what she had done that day.

"It got to the point," she told Tiffany, "that I just dreaded saying I'd been over to the gym. It sounded like I was goofing off while we were stretching our budget to the limit. So for a week or two I stopped going."

Sighing, Betty looked down at her midriff, which had expanded another inch since the last time Tiffany was over. "I've got to go back to moving," Betty vowed.

Tiffany and Betty talked. This time a more confident Betty felt better about asserting her needs. Finally, Betty, with Tiffany's support, came up with a plan—Betty would schedule her exercise routine as if it were a work assignment. She sat down with her husband and explained, friendly but firmly, that her gym visits and the relatively brief time she spent on the exercise bike at home were crucial to her sense of balance. They were a key element that made everything else work properly. These would augment the other commitments in her life—looking for a new job, preparing food, and the cleaning duties she shared with Larry. She insisted she would be responsible for making sure Myron got to classes, and while she was not working, she would deduct her gym fees from the budget she and Larry had earmarked for dining out. Instead of splurging on restaurant meals, she would prepare extra meals at home, and relieve Larry from his Thursday night duty of preparing dinner.

Two weeks later, Betty thanked Tiffany but also took credit herself.

"You know, Tiffany, you gave me the support I needed, but if it hadn't of been for a year of feeling successful with my healthy living plan, I wouldn't have had the confidence to take charge of my life."

CHAPTER NINE

Strategies That Predict Success

S oon, you will begin to navigate life's maze toward success, just like our friends Tiffany, Betty, and their families. We have talked about a lot of issues, scattered a lot of ideas, and crammed in quite a bit. But there is method in our apparent madness, a method that can be broken down into 6 key elements we will summarize in this chapter. Our clients who practice and succeed at these strategies are far more likely to be successful in their Carbohydrate Countdown program, and more important, in their lives in general.

These strategies will also help you control your diabetes (which, by the way, is a great excuse to abstain from temptations. Just tell yourself or your friends that you need to control your glucose). But we want you to think of yourself as healthy. You should be able to succeed at Carbohydrate Countdown without ever bringing into play your medical situation. Think healthy and live healthy! So here are 6 strategies to keep you going and glowing.

Six Strategies for Success

Strategy #1—Monitor your behavior

Observe and record your carbs. (You're already doing that, aren't you?) You should also be keeping tabs on your movements. What you're doing is incredibly simple but powerful. It's based on the premise that people who have a notion of what they're supposed to do are more successful than those who simply wing it. (Think of your records as an instruction sheet, a road map, or in the long view, a ledger.)

Strategy #2—Share your Carbohydrate Countdown

Embarking on the Carbohydrate Countdown journey with a friend or family member is an excellent way to attain long-lasting success. It might help if that friend is a little more advanced at carbohydrate counting and can be a mentor. However, a Carbohydrate Countdown partner who is learning and succeeding at your pace is just fine. It's also good to share with a partner who is newer to Carbohydrate Counting than you. Being a mentor or "Big Sibling" is often a great motivator. In any case, it's much easier to keep up your self-monitoring and your success on the plan if slacking means you have to explain to someone why you're slacking. Plain, good old-fashioned emotional support is always helpful.

Strategy #3—Find your hot buttons

Some things in our life, especially those that seem to occur suddenly, can trigger emotions that can derail us from our best intentions. These are hot buttons. If you identify them, you can turn them around so they can become a benefit rather than an obstacle. How do you recognize a hot button? Think of what happens when a sales clerk pleasantly asks, "Would you like to try on the next size?" What do you do when your mother points out how svelte you *looked* in the wedding picture she keeps prominently displayed? You read how Betty was able to overcome the "hot button" of her husband's insensitivity, automatically triggered whenever she got on an exercise bike. You get the idea. In each of these cases, the strategy involves identifying the hot button and finding a concrete, practical way to avoid or deal with the obstacle.

Strategy #4—Focus on general well-being

Hopefully, you're starting to see how Carbohydrate Countdown coordinates with an overall lifestyle that will allow you to think of yourself more positively. This is easier than you may think. Most of our clients have told us that eating well makes them feel better, which in turn encourages them to exercise. Pretty soon they're sleeping better, which means they're rested, which means they're more effective and successful at work. The cycle continues.

Strategy #5—Manage stress

You need to do this systematically, through exercise and by practicing relaxation techniques. There is a wide menu, so to speak, of opportunities here, many based on exercise principles we've already touched on. Options range from physical activity to more esoteric practices, such as yoga, tai chi, or breathing exercises, which can help you focus specifically on helping your body to relax.

Strategy #6—Social support

"Get a life." Okay, before you think of this advice as callous, imagine that overworked catch phrase as a wake-up call that can help you rally around extracurricular activities; activities that will take your mind off food and weight and help you focus. We have a friend who suggests taking a class—any class. It doesn't matter what the class is (well, maybe a cooking class or anything directly associated with food wouldn't be a good idea at first), as long as you're actively enhancing your knowledge, skills, or talents, as well as interacting with people.

Not All Situations Are Created Equal

Fortunately for our sanity, not all days are the same. We've talked a bit about how to adjust for different types of days—workdays or weekends, for example. Following are some other special situations that require a little creativity to help you stay satisfied and on budget at the same time.

Social situations

This basically breaks down to eating with friends, family, or whoever is going to be both a help and a hindrance in your diet. A dinner with an old friend who looks just as lithe and slender as she did when she was a cheerleader back in high school can be stressful, especially if she's eating enough to feed the whole football team. Keep a sense of humor, but if it's a serious problem, find an alternative. Next time, invite her to join you in a noneating activity.

Social situations don't always have to be difficult, however. If you're having lunch with your Carbohydrate Countdown partner or mentor, you will have an easier time counting carbs than if you were dining alone. Social interaction, as we've mentioned, contributes to reducing stress and offers a sense of well-being that can help your budgeting. You will have to find ways to measure your portions at friends' houses or at restaurants, but this can be accomplished. *Don't become a recluse.* Remember we are on a lifelong eating plan. Just as you learn to cope with your money budget while you're out with friends, you will learn to budget your carbs in any social or business situation.

We don't recommend that you take your measuring arsenal with you to your friend's luncheon. That's why you need to develop that eye for measuring fairly early in the game. The sooner you master this at home where you have measuring cups, spoons, food labels, and other tools to check yourself, the better your eye will become for accurately estimating your CarboUnits visually when you're out and in a hurry.

The biggest pitfall at parties and social situation, of course, is nibbling. If you just can't resist picking up a few potato chips or pretzels as you stroll by the bowl, remember to deduct the munchables from your daily budget.

Desserts require some special strategies. That cheesecake, for example, can be a real challenge, and the choice of how you handle it is yours. If you feel like it, smile pleasantly and refuse. Now that was simple, wasn't it? Maybe not. Remember you do have other choices. Perhaps you may choose to take a few bites, and then deduct a half CarboUnit, or a bit more, depending on how sweet the cake is. You may really enjoy those bites. In fact you may enjoy them more than if you had eaten the whole thing. It might make you feel powerful—you are controlling the food, instead of the reverse (which never makes anyone feel good). Try it, like it, enthuse over it, and tell the host you enjoyed it so much that next time you hope to have more. While it may seem to be rude to leave behind a big hunk of that cheesecake, it's just as rude for a host or hostess to insist that you derail your budget.

Another budgeting technique you can sometimes get away with is bringing some of your own food. This probably won't work well at a black-tie affair, but it will work particularly well with your best friends at informal get-togethers. For example, we have one client who always takes a green salad and dressing to her friends' houses as "a complement to the meal." She relates that usually her friends serve it, and that gives her something to eat and fill her plate, as well as share. That way she can take smaller servings of her friends' rich foods. Do this when you can. Enough said.

The holiday trap

The holidays often bring with them a common pitfall—the holiday blues. This is a difficult season, with parties running from Halloween through Thanksgiving, Christmas, and New Year's, on through those last-minute, start-of-the-year parties some companies tack on to the holiday season. Combine that with the raw weather of the winter, and you have a slowdown in exercise at the same time you're eating more than your share of budget-busting goodies.

To counteract this one-two holiday combo, our hero Tiffany has developed some strategies to help her enjoy a festive season without having to declare diet bankruptcy. These strategies may work for you not only at holiday time, but anytime you are feeling overwhelmed by the need to make food the center of your life.

Let's start with the first shot fired across the bow—Halloween. Like others, this is often the start of the holiday season for Tiffany. Candy pops up everywhere—in her kids' drawers after trick-or-treating, in little jars on her coworkers' desks, on the counter when she leaves the restaurant. For this holiday, Tiffany substitutes an entire meal for one large candy bar. Hardly nutritional nirvana, but that single "goofy" meal won't kill her, either. She figures (and we agree) that one eccentric meal that satisfies her cravings is far better than a candy bar here and a candy bar there for a month or more through the post-Halloween fallout.

And who needs Halloween when Thanksgiving comes so soon afterward?

Tiffany decided she would eat what she wanted for the big Thanksgiving meal that her aunt and cousins prepared. She wouldn't count carbs on that one day. But this wasn't a willy-nilly, plan-busting decision—she had a strategy. Thanksgiving morning Tiffany had a good wholesome breakfast of shredded wheat, nonfat milk, and a half slice of toast with butter. Since dinner was scheduled for about 2 P.M., Tiffany made sure she snacked on some raw carrots—she called them hors d'oeuvres—while everyone else was gorging on potato chips, nuts, and high-calorie snacks. Not only did she avoid the belly-busting snacks, but she also was able to keep her hunger under control. When the big meal came around, she was pleasantly hungry but not famished. Without even thinking about it, she was able to keep her CarboUnits down to a reasonable level. She took seconds on turkey (but just enough gravy to cover her turkey, since she really didn't want to make that meat soggy). And with all that food, who needs bread?

Dessert? Tiffany had 2 of them—she ate the pumpkin pie, and she just had to taste some of Aunt Millie's chocolate cheesecake. "Taste" is the operative word here. She helped herself to a tiny portion. When she saw Aunt Millie, she gushed over how delicious it was, noting how she almost finished eating the whole thing. Then she took one last bite and quietly abandoned the plate.

Having survived Thanksgiving, Tiffany girded herself for the rest of the holidays, including the wave of parties in December given by her friends, her boss, and the civic organizations where she was a member. Clearly, there is a dilemma: This is a time of cheer, a time of socializing. How can she refuse food offered in friendship? Hold on a minute! If her friendships depend on her stuffing herself, maybe she ought to take a look at who her friends are. On the other hand, she didn't want to be confrontational when someone offered her something. So . . . she takes what is offered if she must. Then she eats a bit and leaves the plate somewhere. She figures anyone who is following her around has his or her own problems. But most people aren't so demanding, and Tiffany was able to adopt a 5-point strategy that worked.

1. Tiffany never went to a party on an empty stomach. She had some raw vegetables in a plastic bag in her car, which she munched on *before* she got to the party. As we've said, there's nothing like being ravenously hungry to get you splurging off your budget (and messing up your blood glucose control).

2. A couple of times, Tiffany decided she would splurge. She made sure she had a few extra CarboUnits "banked" by the time she arrived at the Chamber of Commerce Holiday Folk Fest. Tiffany tried the four different kinds of sausage, which she looked forward to each year. Fortunately, they were offered in little bite size bits. She had no excuse not to be dainty. She also had a truffle. But she didn't try to bust her budget by eating mounds of the warm sourdough bread. She had a single piece. But then she told herself that she was over budget, and well, she didn't really need any more bread. Not after that delicious sausage on a sesame cracker.

3. Tiffany kept up her exercise routine. While CarbCounters aren't formally given extra credit for calories burned, Tiffany found that an extra walk with a friend helped keep the rest of her strategy intact—and may have used up an extra CarboUnit here and there. But she didn't (and you shouldn't either) substitute exercise for carbs. Exercise was just a bonus.

4. Tiffany made up her mind to be strong—or at least resolute. She told herself that she didn't have to stuff herself to be polite, and that if anybody said, "Have another piece, dear, it's the holiday," she could politely decline.

5. Tiffany drank lots of mineral water with lemon. This gave her something to do with her hand, and after all, if you're drinking, it's not very dainty to eat. That kept a lot of her friends' from declaring "have another piece."

Restaurant Strategies—More Landmines, More Opportunities

If you're like us, you enjoy eating out and may do it as frequently as possible. During a "time-impaired" workweek, preparing our own meals may take low priority and eating out means we also get to spend quality time talking with our family and friends. However, restaurant eating offers some special challenges, whether it's at the fast-food stand on the corner or the restaurant so fancy, that, as one of our teen-age kids puts it, "They hire a guy who does nothing but write down your name and bring you to the table."

Here are some hints for the CarbCounter looking to survive the woolly restaurant landscape.

Portion control

Portions at restaurants can be a little bit tricky. Usually, the nicer the restaurant, the more sensible the portions are going to be. We're not sure why this is, but it seems the more you pay, the less you get. While it may not be good for your financial budget, this ratio works well for your carb budget. As you move down the ladder, the portions can get more and more out of control. At a place like Applebee's or Denny's, you're usually being served 2 or 3 servings of food at a time. By the time you get to the all-you-can-eat buffet, well, a serving is whatever your brain and your stomach can force down. Fortunately, most chain restaurants are pretty well monitored in order to keep costs down. They may be sliding humongous portions in your face, but there's a good chance they can tell you to the gram how much is on your plate. And it never hurts to ask. Plus, there's an array of books available that give you nutrition information for popular food chains. Having a good idea of how much you're being served is the best way to stay in control and on budget.

The breadbasket

For carbovores, the restaurant breadbasket is a potential trap. Now, for the restaurant, it's a great way to make you feel welcome, and in some cases, encourage you to nibble while you order more drinks. This may be their way of ensuring that after the meal you won't complain because you're still hungry, remembering as you look at the check that the portions weren't quite as large as you might have expected. Go ahead and enjoy the bread, *but remember that it counts on your budget*. More than a token piece or two will probably start adding up to whole CarboUnits. One CarbCounter we know uses the technique of selecting one piece of bread and tearing off small nibble pieces, so it lasts until the entree arrives. Another, after she has decided on the main entree, just keeps an image of that plate in her mind, enabling her to forgo the bread. She knows that delicious pasta is on its way. (She also knows the pasta she ordered is a bit expensive—3 CarboUnits.)

One defensive strategy you CarbCounters may use is to ask your dinner companions to take what they want and then have the wait person remove the breadbasket.

Be assertive

Just because Chef Jacques can't live without the chicken-fat-laden gravy on the turkey, doesn't mean you can't either. You are the customer. Tell the wait person how you want your food. (And remember that cranberry sauce is loaded with carbs—sugar—so if it's the turkey you really want, order it plain, and try the dark meat, which is often not as dry as the white meat.)

Conquering the all-you-can-eat buffet

All-you-can eat restaurants offer special opportunities, as well as special challenges. Since you pick the food, you can control exactly what you get and what you eat. But economics rears its ugly head. *Just because you're paying a single price for "all you can eat," doesn't mean you should feel cheated if you don't stuff yourself.* For some people, an all-you-can-eat restaurant is empowering—for others, it's a diet wrecker. So be sure to approach the line intelligently.

You've probably already noticed that after you pick up your buffet plate, the first food you encounter on the line is the cheapest stuff—lettuce, beans, corn, etc. The restaurant expects you to fill your plate right away, so when you get to the expensive items at the end of the line, there isn't much space left on your plate for the carved roast beef. With this strategy in mind, decide what you want from both ends of the line and pick your portions accordingly. As you can imagine, you will probably want to get most of the food from the beginning of the line. It will save you scads of CarboUnits—unless you drench the lettuce and veggies in high calorie dressing along the way. By focusing on vegetables, the restaurant saves money, and you eat less carbs. It's win-win.

Fast food

Americans spend much of their food dollars in fast food restaurants. The real risk here is not so much a carb meltdown, but a blow to your daily fat allotment. In these places, it's actually pretty hard to pig-out on carbs, because even the carbo-appearing French fries are actually stuffed full of fat. If you're stuck "under the arches" or in the pizza place, try to find the one or two *better* items (which is usually as good as you're going to get), such as the chicken salad. Pizza places sometimes have lower-fat vegetarian pizzas, and many have a salad bar. You will, of course, be faced with the dilemma of sharing (you didn't go to Pizza World by yourself, now, did you?), but some social strategies might be useful. Defer to your guests or hosts on the choice of pizza, nibble off the crusty end of the pizza (lots of yummy carbs you can count as bread), and then take the rest home "for later" or "for the kids." You're strong. You can do it—if you decide to stick to your plan *before* you walk in the restaurant. Don't feel sorry for yourself. Remember you are cementing a great friendship, consummating a great deal, or saving gobs of time for more productive activities later.

Are you getting our message here? We don't think you should feel guilty for eating some of your favorite foods. Just don't forget your budget. You wouldn't buy a new computer every week, but that doesn't mean you shouldn't buy one at all. Further, you wouldn't buy a car that's out of your price range, but by saving and budgeting, you can buy a car that you're happy with. The same goes for your CarboUnit budget. Spending wisely will reap the biggest benefits and the clearest conscience.

Ethnic restaurants

These can offer opportunities as well as landmines. For example, Chinese food has taken a bad rap in recent years for its high concentration of sodium and fat. You can surely go way over your fat allotment. But Chinese restaurants can mesh nicely with Carbohydrate Countdown if you eat like the Chinese traditionally eat. The staple of the diet is rice. (Many Chinese people are shocked that Americans will order several dishes and not even bother to order a rice bowl.) You can eat sensibly keeping in mind that a cup of rice is equivalent to 3 CarboUnits. Then, sparingly order side dishes, trying to select those that contain vegetables. Try to think of the side dishes as a sauce that you spread on the rice. If you use chopsticks, you will likely slow your pace, and that will help keep you satisfied and within your diet budget.

Italian restaurants offer a parallel cultural misunderstanding. Americans seem to think cheese is synonymous with Italian food, but that's wrong. Italian food offers terrific opportunities for serving well-seasoned, healthy vegetables. Choose pasta dishes with a tomato sauce, not the cream sauce (which was traditionally used sparingly). And always remember to visualize portions. Italian restaurants, especially independent ones operated by families, tend to be generous with portions.

Mexican restaurants suffer from the same cultural mistranslation as their Italian counterparts. The abundance of cheese you usually see is a *Norteamericano* adaptation of Mexican food. Mexican families often marvel at how the *Americanos* want cheese with everything. In Mexican restaurants, burritos are often an excellent choice, especially when you tell the server to hold the cheese and sour cream. (By the way, guacamole is a vegetable item that is mostly fat. But it's largely good, monounsaturated fat, and is an excellent choice for your one daily visible portion of fat.)

Breakfasts

One of the authors of this book once sat next to an Indonesian tour guide on a U.S. airliner. The guide marveled at how Americans ate these huge, goofy breakfasts, and in restaurants at least, there didn't seem to be much of an alternative. Actually, most Americans seem to be skipping breakfast more frequently, but for those of you who do think breakfast—at least on some days—we have a few thoughts. First, there is no law that says you have to eat eggs, bacon, pancakes, or waffles at breakfast time. Cereal, cold or hot, is a great choice, and toast with just a bit of jelly is fine, too. True, restaurants often make this choice hard by pricing a bowl of cereal and a glass of orange juice as expensively or even more costly than the "Triple Home Run Breakfast Special" that has meat, eggs, pancakes, and just about everything else but cereal. Here you have to make the choice that sometimes less is more, even if it costs more.

The authors also have another suggestion. When we travel, we usually bring cereal in a plastic bag and in the morning we pick up a small carton of milk. We slice in a banana, heat a cup of the world's most mediocre coffee from the in-room coffee maker, and we're ready to hit a meeting or the hiking trail without having to pick bacon from between our teeth.

Speaking of cereal and milk in the motel . . .

Bringing your own food along whenever possible is a good way to keep your budget under control. Relying on others— hosts or restaurants—for food is a quick and easy way to derail your budget. Sometimes taking control by bringing food is quite easy. Tiffany, for example, found that she could save at least 2 CarboUnits every Saturday by bringing her own can of vegetable juice instead of relying on the donuts, sports drinks, and sugared soda that's usually handed out at her kids' soccer games. Occasionally, just to be sociable, she would bring along a few extra cans of vegetable juice for others, but she rarely found takers. However, a few weeks after starting Carbohydrate Countdown, she found that some of the other parents began bringing their own "grown-up" food choices. Tiffany had started a trend.

Unlike the soccer crowd, gourmet restaurants or even fast food chains tend to frown when you bring in a sack lunch. But sometimes when you join friends, a nice compromise is a deli lunch that you agree to eat at tables outside or in a public location. Then, if you've brought your own food, you can comfortably join in at the table. Some deli owners might even be quite happy to let you bring your own food if you make a token purchase, such as a bottle of mineral water. You might even remind them that the whole group, including those purchasing entire meals, selected the establishment because of their flexible attitude.

Life without meat

Vegetarians can easily enjoy Carbohydrate Countdown. In fact, many of our meatless friends are excellent candidates for Carbohydrate Countdown, because they have unconsciously replaced meat with carbs. Here are a few special hints for people who have chosen to give up meat in favor of a plant-based diet. The protein sources chart (page 52) has several ideas for meatless protein. Just be sure to select portions based on your height.

Naturally, the more flexible you are about defining vegetarian choices, the more protein you have available. But even vegans—those who eat no foods from animal sources—have a number of nutritious and delicious choices from the tofu and peanut butter categories. Vegans and others limiting their intake of animal products should select as many CarboUnits as possible from beans, peas, and lentils to get the protein their bodies need.

CHAPTER TEN

The Joys of Your New Journey

Because overspending your food plan may seem inevitable to you right now, we almost called this section, "Learning to live with failure." That's a little pessimistic, but let's be realistic. You will occasionally vary from the straight and narrow, especially at the beginning. But these lapses won't be fatal to your carb budget if you keep in mind a couple of points.

Look forward

After Tiffany had been on her plan for a week, she met her old girlfriend, Carrie, for coffee. The two long-time friends had a lot of catching up to do. One thing led to another, and they ended up at a pizza parlor, where Tiffany suddenly realized that

1. Carrie's life was so perfect that Tiffany was a bit jealous.
2. Tiffany was hungry.

The end result was that Tiffany ate a whole pepperoni pizza. So what did she do? The same thing we advise you to do when something like this happens. *She got up the next morning as if nothing had happened.* We call this managed denial. We're not telling you it doesn't matter. We are telling you it does matter. But if you want to move forward, forget what happened and start right where you left off.

No excuses

We're going to operate on the assumption that there isn't a single good reason on the planet for you to overspend your budget of CarboUnits. So your husband's car was broadsided by a truck, and your mother brought over some ice cream to make you feel better? Is this okay? No way. We're not telling you that a rational human being wouldn't stray from the straight and narrow under such circumstances. What we are telling you is that it isn't an excuse. Try not to use food here to relieve the stress!

If we sound harsh, that's our loving way of saying that we are trying to make life as unambiguous and as stress-free as possible. And often times you'll find that excuses are more stressful than getting your CarboUnits right in the first place.

If you overspend, (in other words, if you go over your carb budget) just move forward and start the next day as if the lapse had not happened. You'll wake up the second day facing a full carb budget. Some people become so depressed after overeating, that they give up their Carbohydrate Countdown plan altogether. *Don't do that.* If you overspend, muster the resolve to start the next day on target. In the larger scheme of things, that single day of straying won't derail your plan if you return to the program promptly and with renewed dedication.

The Scale Tells All—Eventually

Remember: Don't weigh yourself every day. Once a week is about right. And if you are truly adhering to your diet and you're confident and feeling good about yourself, you might want to just weigh yourself every 2 weeks or so. That will help keep you on track without making you crazy. Remember that the scale is an *indirect* measurement tool. It gives us a benchmark, to be sure, but it doesn't measure health, firmness, or vitality.

As a society, we have an image in our heads where the scale has replaced all other icons. Don't put the scale in the role of making a final judgment. A cartoon once made the point that if scales were automatically set to show weight loss, people would be more motivated and would in fact lose weight. We believe that. Take your Carbohydrate Countdown plan seriously, but don't become a slave to the scale.

Measuring success

I think we can all relate to how Tiffany was able to taste success without submitting to the tyranny of the scale. Not only was she proud of how long-abandoned clothing (or a new two-piece bathing) hugged her body nicely. The compliments from friends made her feel terrific, but the best part of the new Tiffany was the feeling that she was a winner.

Tiffany kept a list of "all of the positive changes I have made." Certainly, being able to fit into a favorite pair of jeans was on that list. Her ability to walk up 3 flights of stairs at work without puffing was on the list. So was her ability to spend the afternoon hiking with her friend Connie without asking that they go back early for a snack.

The most positive news, however, came from Dr. Dillon six months into her Carbohydrate Countdown. The good news was threefold. First, her cholesterol was normal. We can thank her sensible food choices for that. Second, Dr. Dillon was delighted with her weight loss. We can thank her sensible food choices for that, too. In fact, she'd lost 20 pounds. Tiffany hadn't thought to weigh herself for about a week, but she did think that as a successful CarbCounter she was glad she felt so well, could move so well, and could dress so well.

And, third, Dr. Dillon had one more piece of good news.

"Well, Tiffany, it looks as if we don't have to think about diabetes medication just now. Your blood sugar is down to 108, and that's in the normal range (70 to 110 is the normal range). Your test was random, taken 3 hours after you ate, so we would expect this is not the lowest level of blood sugar, which we get after fasting overnight. So just keep on doing what you're doing. No further therapy is required at this time. We'll see you for a check-up in 6 months."

Tiffany couldn't believe her ears.

"That must have been some diet you and Joanne cooked up," said Carla as Tiffany walked out of the office smiling. "I'll bet you have to carry a whole file drawer full of charts and graphs to keep up with things."

Tiffany might have detected a tone of jealousy in Carla's voice, but she was too happy to call her on it.

"No, Carla, I'm following a simple plan I learned with Joanne—Carbohydrate Countdown. By now, it's pretty automatic. Sure, I review my program and notes every once in a while, but mostly it's just become a part of my life."

*   *   *

Despite the angelic smile Tiffany flashed at Carla, we wouldn't want anyone to think that Tiffany had become an angel. The truth is that Tiffany splurges occasionally. Once she went over her daily budget by 4 CarboUnits. She ate a whole pint of extra rich ice cream just after her son's algebra teacher called to say he was flunking and skipping class.

But that night, feeling guilty because of her excess—the flavor of the chocolate swirl with almonds only a distant memory—Tiffany went up to her room. She took out the notebook where all of her successes over the prior 3 months were recorded. One by one, she read off the items that told a world of stories about things that were going right.

One Last Thought–Tiffany Opens Her Closet

There is a secret, dark place where all of our dreams are kept, waiting for the moment when we will return to draw out a past memory. That place is your closet. Yes, your closet contains secrets that even those who live with you are not likely to decode. Let us share with you a story Tiffany told Joanne.

Every week, Tiffany visits her closet, and she was looking forward to a particular visit, really hopeful that she had lost a few pounds since she weighed herself a month earlier.

She had just bought a new silk top, and she knew buried between her father's bowling shirt (she'd inherited that) and the wool sweater she hadn't worn since she spent a winter in Vermont, was a pair of jeans that she hadn't worn for 11 years. A bit retro, the jeans had come the full circle of the fashion loop, a style her friends would find smart but not flashy. Tiffany's 15th high-school reunion was coming up in 2 weeks. She was dying to wear those pants.

Finally, on a Tuesday night after work, just 3 days before the big event, Tiffany entered the darkest reaches of her closet. As she removed the pants her heart pounded almost as hard as at prom night, many years earlier, when a boy whose name she now couldn't quite remember had put his hands gently around her chiffon-covered waist.

Tiffany clumsily dropped the old wire hanger. In her hands were the pants that had remained in the closet for oh-so-many years. She sat on the edge of her bed, spread the pants in front of her, and slowly put her right foot into the proper leg. She stood up and put her left foot through the other leg. With only a dainty jump, she pulled the pants up by the waist, and grabbed for the front button. Tight—you bet—but the pants so long abandoned didn't rip, and they didn't stop short of her belly button. And the button didn't pop. Happier now, Tiffany turned toward the mirror. Not bad. In fact, pretty good.

"Who needs a scale?!"

Carbohydrate Countdown Catalog

Bagels, Breads, Muffins, Tortillas

(1 serving = 1 CarboUnit)	**1 Serving**
Bagel	1/4 (1 oz.)
Biscuit, 2 1/2"	1
Bread, white, whole-wheat, multi-grain	1 slice (1 oz.)
Bread sticks, 4" long × 1/2"	4 (2/3 oz.)
Corn bread, 2" cube	1 (2 oz.)
Croutons	1 cup
English muffin	1/2
Hamburger or hot dog bun	1/2 (1 oz.)
Muffin, small	1 (1/2 oz.)
Pita, 6" across	1/2
Raisin bread	1 slice (1 oz.)
Roll, plain, small	1 (1 oz.)
Stuffing, bread (prepared)	1/3 cup
Taco shell, 6" across	2
Tortilla, corn or flour, 6" across	1

Cereals, Pancakes, Waffles

(1 serving = 1 CarboUnit)	1 Serving
Bran cereals	1/2 cup
Cereals, cooked	1/2 cup
Cereals, unsweetened, ready-to-eat	3/4 cup
Granola	1/4 cup
Grape-Nuts	1/4 cup
Grits, cooked	1/2 cup
Muesli	1/4 cup
Oats, cooked	1/2 cup
Pancakes, 4" across	1
Puffed cereal	1 1/2 cups
Shredded Wheat	1/2 cup
Waffle, 4 1/2" square	1

Grains, Pasta, Potatoes, Rice

(1 serving = 1 CarboUnit)	1 Serving
Bulgur, cooked	1/2 cup
Corn	1/2 cup
Corn-on-the-cob	1/2 cob (5 oz.)
Couscous, cooked	1/3 cup
French-fried potatoes	16 (3 oz.)
Kasha, cooked	1/2 cup
Millet, cooked	1/3 cup
Pasta, spaghetti, and noodles, cooked	1/3 cup
Polenta (corn meal), cooked	1/2 cup
Potato, baked or boiled	1 small (3 oz.)
Potato, mashed	1/2 cup
Rice, white or brown, cooked	1/3 cup
Yam or sweet potato	1/2 cup

Chips, Crackers, Snacks

(1 serving = 1 CarboUnit)	1 Serving
Crackers, round type	6
Graham crackers, 2 1/2" square	3
Matzoh	3/4 oz.
Melba toast	4 slices
Oyster crackers	24
Popcorn, plain	3 cups
Potato chips	15–20 (3/4 oz.)
Pretzels	3/4 oz.
Rice cakes, 4" across	2
Saltine-type crackers	6
Tortilla chips	10 (1 oz.)

Vegetables (cooked, canned, or frozen)

(1 serving = 1 CarboUnit)	**1 Serving**
Artichoke	1 medium
Artichoke hearts, canned in water	3/4 cup
Asparagus	18 spears, 1 1/2 cups
Baked beans	1/3 cup
Beans (green, wax, Italian)	1 1/2 cups
Beans and peas (garbanzo, pinto, kidney, white, split, black-eyed)	1/2 cup
Beets	1 cup
Broccoli	1 1/2 cups
Brussels sprouts	1 cup
Cabbage	1 1/2 cups
Carrots	1 cup, 2 med. raw
Cauliflower	1 1/2 cups
Eggplant	1 1/2 cups
Greens (collard, kale, mustard, chard, turnip)	1 1/2 cups
Leeks	1 1/2 cups
Lentils	1/2 cup
Lima beans	2/3 cup
Mixed vegetables with corn or peas	1 cup
Mushrooms	1 1/2 cups
Okra	1 1/2 cups
Peas, green	1/2 cup
Sauerkraut	1 1/2 cups
Spinach	1 1/2 cups
Squash, summer	1 1/2 cups
Squash, winter (acorn, butternut)	1 cup
Tomato, cooked or canned	1 cup
Tomato/vegetable juice	1 1/2 cups
Turnips	1 1/2 cups
Water chestnuts	1 cup
Zucchini	1 1/2 cups

Salad Vegetables (raw)

(2 cups raw mix = 1/2 CarboUnit)

Bean sprouts	Onion
Cabbage	Parsley
Celery	Peppers
Cucumber	Radish
Endive	Romaine lettuce
Green onions	Spinach
Lettuce	

Milk, Soy Milk, and Yogurt

(1 serving = 1 CarboUnit)	**1 Serving**
Chocolate milk, reduced-fat	1/2 cup
Fruit-flavored yogurt, with artificial sweetener	2/3 cup (6 oz.)
Lactose-reduced milk	1 cup
Milk, non-fat, 1%, or reduced-fat	1 cup
Rice milk	1 cup
Soy milk, flavored	1 cup
Yogurt, plain	3/4 cup

Fruits, Fruit Juice

(1 serving = 1 CarboUnit)	1 Serving
Apple, dried	4 rings
Apple juice/cider	1/2 cup
Applesauce	1/2 cup
Apple, small	1 (4 oz.)
Apricots, canned	1/2 cup
Apricots, fresh or dried	4 whole, 8 halves
Banana, small	1 (4 oz.)
Blackberries	3/4 cup
Blueberries	3/4 cup
Cherries, canned	1/2 cup
Cherries, fresh	12 (3 oz.)
Cranberry juice cocktail	1/3 cup
Dates	3 medium
Figs, fresh or dried	2 medium
Fruit cocktail	1/2 cup
Fruit juice blends, 100% juice	1/3 cup
Grapefruit	1/2
Grapefruit juice	1/2 cup
Grapefruit sections, canned	3/4 cup
Grape juice	1/3 cup
Grapes, small	17 (3 oz.)
Kiwi	1
Lemonade	1/2 cup
Mandarin oranges	3/4 cup
Mango, small	1/2 fruit
Melons (cantaloupe, honeydew, watermelon)	1 cup cubes
Nectarine, small	1 (5 oz.)
Orange juice	1/2 cup
Orange, small	1 (6 1/2 oz.)
Papaya	1/2 fruit, 1 cup cubes
Peach, medium	1 (4 oz.)

Fruits, Fruit Juice (*Continued*)

(1 serving = 1 CarboUnit)	1 Serving
Peaches, canned	1/2 cup
Pear, canned	1/2 cup
Pear, small	1
Pineapple, canned	1/2 cup
Pineapple, fresh	3/4 cup
Pineapple juice	1/2 cup
Plums	2
Plums, canned	1/2 cup
Prune juice	1/3 cup
Prunes, dried	3
Raisins	2 Tbsp.
Raspberries	1 cup
Strawberries (whole berries)	1 1/4 cups
Tangerines	2 (8 oz.)

Desserts, Sweets

(1 serving = 1 CarboUnit)	1 Serving
Animal crackers	8
Brownie, unfrosted	2" square
Cake	2" square
Cookie	2 small
Cranberry sauce	1/4 cup
Fruit juice bars, frozen	1 bar (3 oz.)
Gingersnaps	3
Granola bar	1 bar
Ice cream	1/2 cup
Jam or jelly	1 Tbsp.
Sherbet, sorbet	1/2 cup
Soda, regular	5 oz.
Syrup, regular	1 Tbsp.
Vanilla wafers	5
Yogurt, frozen	1/3 cup

(1 serving = 2 CarboUnits)	1 Serving
Doughnut, glazed	1 medium (2 oz.)
Doughnut, plain cake	1 medium (1 1/2 oz.)
Pie, fruit or custard	1/8 pie
Sweet roll or Danish	1 (2 1/2 oz.)

*adapted from: Exchange Lists for Weight Management. 2003. American Diabetes Association, Inc./American Dietetic Association.

Sample Menus

Based on height and height alone

Height 5 ft.   165 Carbohydrate (Carb) grams   11.0 CarboUnits

Time	CarboUnit Goal & Food	Carb g	CarboUnits
Morning	2 CarboUnits		
	Corn tortilla, one	15.0	1.0
	Mozzarella cheese, 1 slice		
	Mango pieces, 1/2 cup	15.0	1.0
	Coffee		
Mid-Day	3.5 CarboUnits		
	Noodle soup, 1 1/2 cups, with	30.0	2.0
	2 ounces chicken and		
	3/4 cup of carrots and celery	7.0	0.5
	Whole grain crackers or saltines, 6	15.0	1.0
	Sparkling water		
Afternoon	1.0 CarboUnit		
	Gingersnaps, 3	15.0	1.0
Evening	3.5 CarboUnits		
	Beef or Pork, 3 ounces, in		
	Stir-fry with 3/4 cup mixed		
	green pepper, onions, & cabbage	7.0	0.5
	2 tsp. olive oil		
	Steamed white or brown rice, 2/3 cup	30.0	2.0
	1 cup 1% milk	15.0	1.0
	Tea		
Bedtime	1.0 CarboUnit		
	Tangerine, 2	15.0	1.0
DAY'S TOTAL		**165.0**	**11.0**

Height 5 ft. 1 in.   170 Carbohydrate (Carb) grams   11.5 CarboUnits

Time	CarboUnit Goal & Food	Carb g	CarboUnits
Morning	2 CarboUnits		
	Whole wheat English muffin, one	30.0	2.0
	Cottage cheese, 1/4 cup		
	Small spoonful of butter		
	Coffee		
Mid-Day	3.5 CarboUnits		
	Sandwich with 2 slices multigrain bread and 1 ounces turkey and 1 ounce Swiss cheese	30.0	2.0
	Small spoonful mayonnaise, lettuce and tomato slice		
	Dill pickle spear(s)		
	Potato chips, 20 chips	22.0	1.5
	Sparkling water		
Afternoon	1.0 CarboUnit		
	Grapes, 17	15.0	1.0
Evening	4.0 CarboUnits		
	Lamb chop, 3 ounces broiled		
	Small red potatoes, 2	15.0	1.0
	Small spoonful of butter		
	Winter squash, 1 cup	15.0	1.0
	Fresh orange, one	15.0	1.0
	1 cup 1% milk	15.0	1.0
	Tea		
Bedtime	1.0 CarboUnit		
	Popcorn, 3 cups	15.0	1.0
DAY'S TOTAL		170.0	11.5

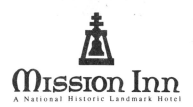

Mission Inn
A National Historic Landmark Hotel

Monica McCorkle

381

3649 Mission Inn Avenue, Riverside, California 92501
(909) 784-0300 • FAX (909) 683-1342
Reservations (800) 843-7755
www.missioninn.com

Height 5 ft. 2 in.   180 Carbohydrate (Carb) grams   12.0 CarboUnits

Time	CarboUnit Goal & Food	Carb g	CarboUnits
Morning	2 CarboUnits		
	1 Pancake, 4"	15.0	1.0
	Small spoonful of butter		
	Applesauce with cinnamon, 1/2 cup	15.0	1.0
	Coffee		
Mid-Day	3.5 CarboUnits		
	Salad greens with 1/4 cup tuna and		
	1 small potato and	15.0	1.0
	3/4 cup green beans	7.0	0.5
	Black olives, 5		
	1 soup spoon salad dressing		
	Whole wheat pita bread, one	30.0	2.0
	Iced tea		
Afternoon	1.5 CarboUnits		
	Berries, 1/2 cup	7.0	0.5
	1 cup 1% milk	15.0	1.0
Evening	4.0 CarboUnits		
	Pasta,1 cup, with a	30.0	2.0
	3-ounce chicken breast		
	Small spoonful of olive oil and		
	1/2 cup cooked tomato with onion		
	and garlic	7.0	0.5
	French bread, 2 small slices	15.0	1.0
	Grapes, 8	7.0	0.5
	Tea		
Bedtime	1.0 CarboUnit		
	Frozen fruit juice bar	15.0	1.0
DAY'S TOTAL		180.0	12.0

Height 5 ft. 3 in.   190 Carbohydrate (Carb) grams   12.5 CarboUnits

Time	CarboUnit Goal & Food	Carb g	CarboUnits
Morning	2.5 CarboUnits		
	Oatmeal, 1/2 cup cooked with	15.0	1.0
	Raisins, 1 soup spoon	7.0	0.5
	1 cup 1% milk	15.0	1.0
	Coffee		
Mid-Day	3.5 CarboUnits		
	3 ounce hamburger on whole bun with Lettuce, tomato, & dill pickle slices	30.0	2.0
	Small spoon of mayonnaise		
	French Fried potatoes, 10 spears	7.0	0.5
	Apple, one sliced	15.0	1.0
	Sparkling water		
Afternoon	1.5 CarboUnits		
	Cookies, 2 small	15.0	1.0
	Coffee Latte with 1/2 cup 1% milk	7.0	0.5
Evening	4.0 CarboUnits		
	Salmon, 3 ounces broiled		
	Couscous, 2/3 cup cooked	30.0	2.0
	Salad greens with tomato & cucumber	7.0	0.5
	One soupspoon salad dressing		
	Brussels sprouts, 1/2 cup	7.0	0.5
	Pear, one	15.0	1.0
	Tea		
Bedtime	1.0 CarboUnit		
	Ice cream, 1/2 cup	15.0	1.0
DAY'S TOTAL		190.0	12.5

Height 5 ft. 4 in.   195 Carbohydrate (Carb) grams   13.0 CarboUnits

Time	CarboUnit Goal & Food	Carb g	CarboUnits
Morning	2.5 CarboUnits		
	English muffin, one, with	30.0	2.0
	Cheddar cheese, melted		
	Cantaloupe cubes, 1/2 cup	15.0	1.0
	Coffee		
Mid-Day	3.5 CarboUnits		
	Tomato soup, 1 cup	15.0	1.0
	Tuna Fish, 1/4 cup, sandwich with		
	lettuce and whole wheat bread, 2 slices	30.0	2.0
	Small spoon of mayonnaise		
	1/4 cup apple juice in	7.0	0.5
	Sparkling water		
Afternoon	1.5 CarboUnits		
	Low-fat plain yogurt, 1 cup, topped with	15.0	1.0
	Banana, 1/2 small	7.0	0.5
Evening	4.0 CarboUnits		
	Roast beef, 3 ounces		
	Steamed potatoes, 2 small (1 cup)	30.0	2.0
	Carrots, 1 cup cooked	15.0	1.0
	Spinach salad		
	One soupspoon salad dressing		
	Frozen fruit juice bar	15.0	1.0
	Iced tea		
Bedtime	1.5 CarboUnits		
	Muffin, 1 medium	22.0	1.5
DAY'S TOTAL		195.0	13.0

Height 5 ft. 5 in.   400 Carbohydrate (Carb) grams   13.5 CarboUnits

Time	CarboUnit Goal & Food	Carb g	CarboUnits
Morning	2.5 CarboUnits		
	Multi-grain bread, toasted, 1 slice	15.0	1.0
	Small spoonful of butter		
	Low-fat yogurt, 1/2 cup	7.0	0.5
	Peach slices, fresh or canned 1/2 cup	15.0	1.0
	Coffee		
Mid-Day	4.0 CarboUnits		
	Tacos with 2 corn tortilla shells	30.0	2.0
	1/4 cup cooked ground beef or diced cooked chicken		
	Grated Monterey Jack cheese, 3 tablespoons		
	Chopped tomatoes, onions, and peppers, generous		
	Red tomato salsa		
	1/2 cup lemonade in sparkling water	15.0	1.0
	Pineapple, fresh or canned, 1/2 cup	15.0	1.0
Afternoon	1.5 CarboUnits		
	Trail mix: 2 tablespoons of raisins, dried apricot halves (4) diced, and one soup spoon of nuts	22.0	1.5
Evening	4.0 CarboUnits		
	Lamb chop, 3 ounces		
	One small spoon of mint jelly	15.0	1.0
	Mashed potatoes, 3/4 cup	22.0	1.5
	Artichoke, cooked	7.0	0.5
	Lemon butter for dipping		
	Mixed green salad		
	One soupspoon salad dressing		
	Whole grain roll	15.0	1.0
	Coffee		
Bedtime	1.5 CarboUnits		
	1 cup 1% milk	15.0	1.0
	Cookie, one small	7.0	0.5
DAY'S TOTAL		200.0	13.5

Note: header says "200 Carbohydrate (Carb) grams".

Height 5 ft. 6 in.   210 Carbohydrate (Carb) grams   14.0 CarboUnits

Time	CarboUnit Goal & Food	Carb g	CarboUnits
Morning	3.0 CarboUnits		
	2 Multigrain waffles, 4"	30.0	2.0
	Small spoonful of butter		
	Two small spoons of syrup	15.0	1.0
	Coffee		
Mid-Day	4.0 CarboUnits		
	Chicken salad, 1/3 cup, in		
	Whole wheat pita bread with	30.0	2.0
	Shredded lettuce		
	Fresh peppers, sliced, and cherry tomatoes		
	Papaya, sliced, 1/2 cup	15.0	1.0
	1 cup 1% milk	15.0	1.0
Afternoon	1.5 CarboUnits		
	Applesauce, 3/4 cup	22.0	1.5
Evening	4.0 CarboUnits		
	Salmon, 3 ounces broiled		
	White or brown rice, 2/3 cup	30.0	2.0
	Lima beans, 2/3 cup	15.0	1.0
	Small spoon of butter		
	Ice cream, 1/2 cup	15.0	1.0
	Tea		
Bedtime	1.5 CarboUnits		
	Pear, large	22.0	1.5
	Cheese slices, 2		
DAY'S TOTAL		210.0	14.0

Height 5 ft. 7 in.   220 Carbohydrate (Carb) grams   14.5 CarboUnits

Time	CarboUnit Goal & Food	Carb g	CarboUnits
Morning	3.0 CarboUnits		
	Bran muffin, medium	22.0	1.5
	Small spoonful of butter		
	Whole grapefruit, sectioned	22.0	1.5
	Coffee		
Mid-Day	4.0 CarboUnits		
	Chef salad with sliced turkey, Swiss cheese, 1 hard cooked egg, tomato wedges and plenty of salad greens		
	One soupspoon of salad dressing		
	Rye bread, 2 slices	30.0	2.0
	Melon, 1 cup cubed	15.0	1.0
	1 cup 1% milk	15.0	1.0
Afternoon	2.0 CarboUnits		
	Frozen yogurt or fruit smoothie, 2/3 cup	30.0	2.0
Evening	4.0 CarboUnits		
	Soybean curd (tofu), firm, 3/4 cup, with soy sauce and onions, green beans, and celery	7.0	0.5
	Soba noodles, 1 cup	30.0	2.0
	Snow peas, steamed, generous	7.0	0.5
	Fresh orange, one sectioned	15.0	1.0
	Tea		
Bedtime	1.5 CarboUnits		
	Ready-to-eat cereal mix with nuts, 1 cup	22.0	1.5
DAY'S TOTAL		220.0	14.5

Height 5 ft. 8 in.   230 Carbohydrate (Carb) grams   15.0 CarboUnits

Time	CarboUnit Goal & Food	Carb g	CarboUnits
Morning	3.0 CarboUnits		
	Cinnamon bread, 2 slices	30.0	2.0
	Small spoonful of cream cheese		
	Low-fat yogurt, 1/2 cup with	7.0	0.5
	Blueberries, 2/3 cup	7.0	0.5
	Coffee		
Mid-Day	4.0 CarboUnits		
	Lentil soup, 1 cup	30.0	2.0
	Corn bread, 2" cube	15.0	1.0
	Mixed fresh fruit salad, 3/4 cup	15.0	1.0
	Iced tea		
Afternoon	2.0 CarboUnits		
	Granola bar	30.0	2.0
Evening	4.0 CarboUnits		
	Halibut, 3 ounces, baked with tomatoes, onions, and olives		
	Bulgur, cooked, 1/2 cup	15.0	1.0
	Broccoli spears	7.0	0.5
	6 Breadsticks, 4" long	22.0	1.5
	Plums, 2 whole	15.0	1.0
	Sparkling water		
Bedtime	2.0 CarboUnits		
	Chocolate pudding, 1/2 cup	30.0	2.0
DAY'S TOTAL		230.0	15.0

Height 5 ft. 9 in.   235 Carbohydrate (Carb) grams   15.5 CarboUnits

Time	CarboUnit Goal & Food	Carb g	CarboUnits
Morning	3.0 CarboUnits		
	Scrambled eggs, 2, with chopped vegetables		
	Small spoonful of olive oil		
	Bagel	30.0	2.0
	Orange juice, 1/2 cup	15.0	1.0
	Coffee		
Mid-Day	4.0 CarboUnits		
	Sliced turkey, 2 ounces on		
	Whole wheat bread, 2 slices	30.0	2.0
	With cranberry sauce, one soup spoon	7.0	0.5
	One small spoon of mayonnaise		
	Potato chips, 8	7.0	0.5
	1 cup 1% milk	15.0	1.0
Afternoon	2.5 CarboUnits		
	Pear, one sliced	15.0	1.0
	Figs, 3 dried	15.0	1.0
	Dates, 2 small	7.0	0.5
	Cheddar cheese, 1 oz.		
Evening	4.0 CarboUnits		
	Pork tenderloin, 3 ounces with		
	Bread stuffing, 2/3 cup	30.0	2.0
	Sweet potato, 1/2 cup baked	15.0	1.0
	Apple, 1 diced, and walnut salad on		
	lettuce leaf	15.0	1.0
	One small spoon of mayonnaise		
	Iced tea		
Bedtime	2.0 CarboUnits		
	Popcorn, 3 cups	15.0	1.0
	Lemonade, 1/2 cup, with sparkling water	15.0	1.0
DAY'S TOTAL		235.0	15.5

Height 5 ft. 10 in.   245 Carbohydrate (Carb) grams   16.5 CarboUnits

Time	CarboUnit Goal & Food	Carb g	CarboUnits
Morning	3.0 CarboUnits		
	Ready-to-eat cereal, 3/4 cup , with	15.0	1.0
	Blueberries, 3/4 cup	15.0	1.0
	1 cup 1% milk	15.0	1.0
	Coffee		
Mid-Day	4.0 CarboUnits		
	Taco salad with tortilla chips, 15, with	30.0	2.0
	Mixed greens and ground beef, 2 oz.,		
	and black beans 1/2 cup	15.0	1.0
	Fresh tomato salsa		
	Papaya cubes, 1 cup	15.0	1.0
	Sparkling water		
Afternoon	2.5 CarboUnits		
	Whole wheat crackers, 7, with	22.0	1.5
	Peanut Butter, one soup spoon		
	1 cup 1% milk	15.0	1.0
Evening	4.0 CarboUnits		
	Beef stew, 3 ounces, with 1/2 cup carrots		
	and onions	7.0	0.5
	Red potatoes, 2 small	15.0	1.0
	French bread, 2 slices	30.0	2.0
	Green beans, 3/4 cup	7.0	0.5
	Tea		
Bedtime	3.0 CarboUnits		
	2 Brownies, 2" square	30.0	2.0
	1/2 cup 1% milk	15.0	1.0
DAY'S TOTAL		245.0	16.5

References and Resources

American Diabetes Association. Evidence-based nutrition principles and recommendations for the treatment and prevention of diabetes and related complications: position statement. *Diabetes Care* 2002;25(suppl 1):S50–S60.

Diabetes Prevention Program Research Group. Reduction in the incidence of type 2 diabetes with lifestyle intervention or metformin. *New England Journal of Medicine* 2002;346:393–403.

Exchange Lists for Meal Planning. American Diabetes Association and the American Dietetic Association. 2003.

The Diabetes Carbohydrate and Fat Gram Guide, 2nd Edition. Holzmeister, LA. American Diabetes Association and the American Dietetic Association. 2000

Foreyt JP, Goodrick GK. Attributes of successful approaches to weight loss and control. *Applied & Preventive Psychology* 1994;3:209–215.

Franz MJ, Bantle JP, Beebe CA, et al. Evidence-based nutrition principles and recommendations for the treatment and prevention of diabetes and related complications: technical review. *Diabetes Care* 2002;25:148–198.

Inside the Brain. Kotulak R. Andrews McMeel Publishing. 1996.

Complete Guide to Carb Counting. Warshaw HS, Kulkarni K. American Diabetes Association. 2001.

The Diabetes Food and Nutrition Bible. Warshaw HS, Webb R. American Diabetes Association. 2001.

Internet Resource with helpful links:

American Diabetes Association, *www.diabetes.org*, Consumer information includes *Basic Diabetes Information*; *Type 2 Diabetes*; *Community and Resources*, which gives specific state information; and a link to health insurance legislation. Recipes, nutrition information, and exercise information also available.

American Dietetics Association, *www.eatright.org*, offers a variety of links and information on sound nutrition. Click on the healthy lifestyle icon at the site for news and tips on good health and eating.

National Heart, Lung and Blood Institute's Healthy Weight Project, *http://www.nhlbi.nih.gov/health/public/heart/obesity/lose_wt/index.htm* offers a Body Mass Index (BMI) calculator and a variety of information.

National Library of Medicine, MEDLINEplus Health Information, Diabetes, *www.nlm.nih.gov/medlineplus/diabetes.html*

United States Department of Agriculture (USDA), *www.health.gov/dietaryguidelines/*, Dietary guidelines for Americans.

Index

About the American Diabetes Association

The American Diabetes Association is the nation's leading voluntary health organization supporting diabetes research, information, and advocacy. Its mission is to prevent and cure diabetes and to improve the lives of all people affected by diabetes. The American Diabetes Association is the leading publisher of comprehensive diabetes information. Its huge library of practical and authoritative books for people with diabetes covers every aspect of self-care—cooking and nutrition, fitness, weight control, medications, complications, emotional issues, and general self-care.

To order American Diabetes Association books: Call 1-800-232-6733. Or log on to http://store.diabetes.org

To join the American Diabetes Association: Call 1-800-806-7801. www.diabetes.org/membership

For more information about diabetes or ADA programs and services: Call 1-800-342-2383. E-mail: Customerservice@diabetes.org or log on to www.diabetes.org

To locate an ADA/NCQA Recognized Provider of quality diabetes care in your area: www.ncqa.org/dprp/

To find an ADA Recognized Education Program in your area: Call 1-888-232-0822. www.diabetes.org/recognition/education.asp

To join the fight to increase funding for diabetes research, end discrimination, and improve insurance coverage: Call 1-800-342-2383. www.diabetes.org/advocacy

To find out how you can get involved with the programs in your community: Call 1-800-342-2383. See below for program Web addresses.

- *American Diabetes Month:* Educational activities aimed at those diagnosed with diabetes—month of November. www.diabetes.org/ADM
- *American Diabetes Alert:* Annual public awareness campaign to find the undiagnosed—held the fourth Tuesday in March. www.diabetes.org/alert
- *The Diabetes Assistance & Resources Program (DAR):* diabetes awareness program targeted to the Latino community. www.diabetes.org/DAR
- *African American Program:* diabetes awareness program targeted to the African American community. www.diabetes.org/africanamerican
- *Awakening the Spirit: Pathways to Diabetes Prevention & Control:* diabetes awareness program targeted to the Native American community. www.diabetes.org/awakening

To find out about an important research project regarding type 2 diabetes: www.diabetes.org/ada/research.asp

To obtain information on making a planned gift or charitable bequest: Call 1-888-700-7029. www.diabetes.org/ada/plan.asp

To make a donation or memorial contribution: Call 1-800-342-2383. www.diabetes.org/ada/cont.asp